SCENE SIZE-UP

- Stabilize scene before moving on.
- Call for specialized teams as needed.
- Danger can be immediate or can be slow in developing, such as darkness, weather, tides, etc.

DANGER:
- Is the scene safe to enter?
- The four priorities:
    1. personal
    2. partner
    3. public
    4. patient

MECHANISM OF INJURY:
- What type of forces involved?
- Distance of fall, type of landing?
- Mechanism of injury to spine?
    - positive
    - uncertain
    - negative

NUMBERS:
- Determine number of victims.
- Account for everyone.
- Determine need for more rescuers.

INITIAL ASSESSMENT-4

INITIAL ASSESSMENT
GENERAL RULES

The initial assessment is a quick look at urgent problems in the body's Critical Systems: Respiratory, Circulatory, Nervous.

- **Stop and fix problems as you find them.**
- **Even if you do everything right, some people still die.**
- **Air goes in and out, blood goes round and round, and oxygen is good.**

COMPONENT	ASSESSMENT	TREATMENT
AIRWAY		

Is air moving in and out?	• *FOREIGN BODY*
	  - cork
		• look for obstruction
		• ventilate
		• "POP" cork
		  (abdominal thrusts)

NO →	• *FLUID* - blood, water, vomit	• gravity/suction
YES	• *POSITION* - kinked	• traction in position • jaw thrust

	• *SWELLING*
	  - trauma, burns,
	    anaphylaxis
		• BLS/ALS
		• Treat cause if possible

COMPONENT	ASSESSMENT	TREATMENT

BREATHING

Adequate?

- trauma?
- medical?
- environmental?

- **P**osition of comfort
- **R**eassurance
- **O**2 100% if available
- **P**ositive pressure ventilation (PPV)

NO →

YES ↓

- inspection
- palpation
- auscultation
- rate/effort

PROP ←

- treat underlying cause if possible
- BLS/ALS

CIRCULATION

Pulse/Perfusion?

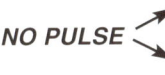

NO PULSE → CPR/ALS
or
DO NOT RESUSCITATE

NO →

YES ↓

INADEQUATE PERFUSION

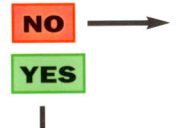

- ▼ distal pulses
- ▼ AVPU
- skin

- treat cause if possible
- ALS, ASAP
- P.R.O.P.

SEVERE BLEEDING

NO **YES** →

- gloves
- find bleeder(s)
- well aimed direct pressure
- elevation
- ? pressure points
- ? tourniquet

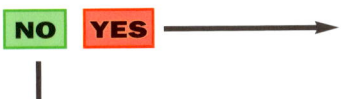

INITIAL ASSESSMENT-5

INITIAL ASSESSMENT-6

COMPONENT	ASSESSMENT	TREATMENT

NERVOUS

Mechanism for spine injury?

YES or UNCLEAR →

- no unnecessary movement
- protect spine
- hands on stabilization

- Assess further in focused assessment

NO ↓

Level of Consciousness Awake / Alert?

AVPU ↓

NO → *Awake*: further define mental status
Verbal: does the patient respond to verbal stimulus
Pain: does the patient respond to painful stimulus
Unresponsive: totally unconscious

YES

- There is no specific treatment
- ALS/BLS?

- If <A, there may be an evolving circulatory, respiratory, or nervous system problem.

MOVE ON TO FOCUSED ASSESSMENT

Emergency roll for the potentially spine injured patient (one rescuer)

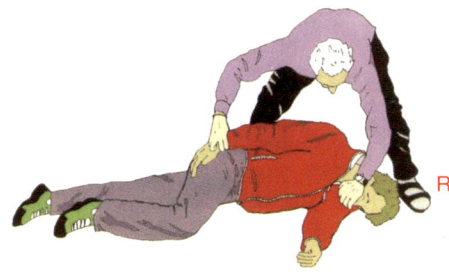

- Checking the Critical Systems
Circulation (pulse and bleeding)
Respiration (airway and breathing)
Nervous (AVPU and spine)

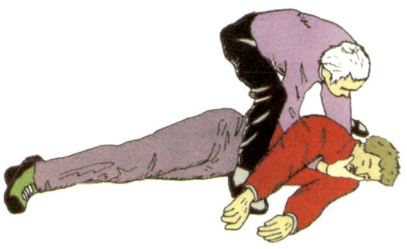

- Vise-locking the spine - support the head and spinal column by grasping the jaw and back of head and squeeze the centerline of the body between forearms.

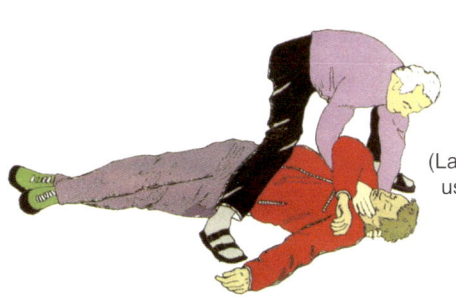

- Roll the patient onto his back. (Larger patients may require you to use the heel of your foot to nudge the patient's pelvis into rolling along with the upper body).

RESPIRATORY SYSTEM - 7

RESPIRATORY SYSTEM - 8

**Emergency roll for the potentially spine injured patient to clear airway
(one rescuer)**

• Support the patient's head and neck with one hand and reach around to center of back with the other.

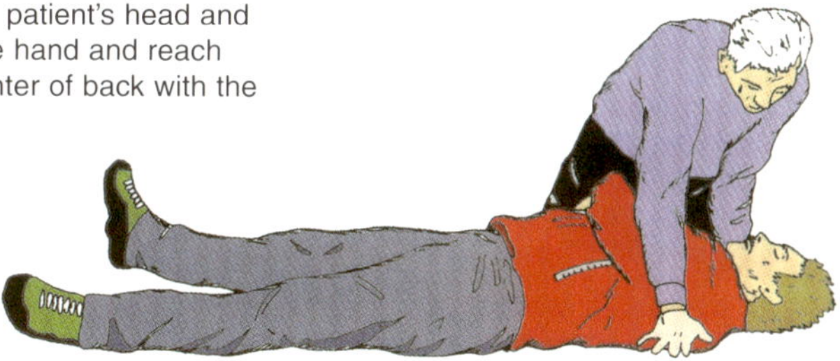

• While supporting the patient's head and neck, roll patient onto your thighs and clear airway.

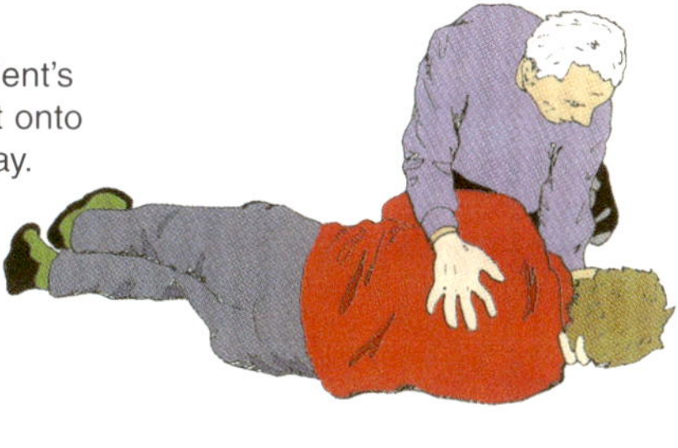

BLS/ALS TREATMENT PROTOCOLS

Normothermic Patient
(> 90°F, 32°C)

Do NOT BEGIN Resuscitation:
- obviously dead, lethal injuries
- submerged under H2O greater than 1 hour
- blunt trauma* with no pulse/breathing
- DNR orders
    - * some EMS protocols

START BLS/ALS OTHERWISE

WHEN TO STOP:
- Patient recovers
- Authorized medical professional pronounces patient dead
- Transfer to other resources
- Rescuers exhausted OR at risk

WILDERNESS CONTEXT:

NORMOTHERMIC PATIENT
- Stop CPR after sustained cardiopulmonary arrest (> 30 continuous minutes).

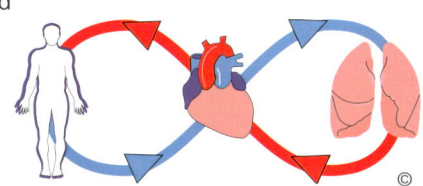

CPR SUMMARY-10

CPR SUMMARY

1. Check consciousness
2. Call EMS (if possible)
3. Open airway
4. Look, Listen, Feel

Give breaths

BREATHS DON'T GO IN

Reposition

Try again → **YES**

NO

Thrusts and sweep

BREATHS GO IN

Check Pulse

NO   **YES**

Chest compressions & ventilations

Ventilations only

Reassess Periodically

TIME TO CPR	SURVIVAL PERCENTAGES*			
	TIME TO ACLS (minutes)			
(minutes)	0 - 8	8 - 16	16+	>30
0 - 4	43%	19%	10%	0%
4 - 8	26%	19%	5%	0%
8 - 12	N.A.	6%	0%	0%

*Adapted from Eisenberg

FOCUSED ASSESSMENT
(MEDICAL vs TRAUMA)

The speed, detail and order of the focused assessment is variable. Complete the assessment, prioritize the problem list; then treat the problems.

EXAM:
- examine problem areas
- compare to "the good side"
- how does it look? How does it feel?
- check Range of Motion (ROM) and Circulation, Sensation, Motor (CSM)

HISTORY:
- *SYMPTOMS*
- *ALLERGIES* - to what? how severe?
- *MEDICATIONS* - what for? compliant? OTC / Rx?
- *PAST HISTORY* - significant medical history
- *LAST* - food and fluid intake; menstrual cycle
- *EVENTS* - detailed description

VITAL SIGNS:
- *PULSE* - rate per minute (normal adult 60-100 beats/min.)
- *RESPIRATIONS* - rate/min. (normal adult 12-20/min), effort
- *BLOOD PRESSURE* - systolic/diastolic
- *SKIN* - color, temperature, moisture
- *TEMPERATURE* - core temperature
- *AVPU* - mental status, level of consciousness, (consider STOPEATS, pg.21)

SOAP FORMATTING-12

SOAP FORMATTING

SUBJECTIVE: scene, story, symptoms and history
OBJECTIVE: exam findings, vital signs

ASSESSMENT (problems)	ANTICIPATED PROBLEMS	PLAN (treatment)
1		
2		
3		
4		

RADIO SOAP

S This is . . . to . . . (location, situation)
We have a . . . (story, MOI, history of events)
Patient is complaining of . . . (symptoms)

O On exam we found . . . (tenderness, CSM, ROM)
Vital signs are . . .

A Our problem list includes . . .

A' Anticipated problems . . .

P Our plan is . . . request . . .
Next contact, etc. . . .

SOAP NOTE

SCENE

SUBJECTIVE

S Symptoms

A Allergies
M Medications
P Past History
L Last Meal
E Events

OBJECTIVE

EXAM:

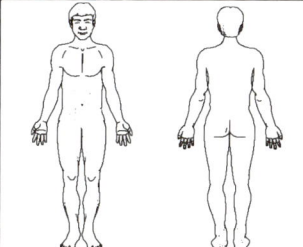

VITAL SIGNS

Time	Pulse	Resp.	B/P	Skin	Temp.	AVPU
			/			
			/			
			/			
			/			
			/			
			/			
			/			

Emergency training for outdoor professionals.™

207-665-2707 888-WILD-MED 189 Dudley Road, Bryant Pond, ME 04219 © WMA, INC 1995

ASSESSMENT AND TREATMENT PLAN

A = Assessment (Problem List)	A' = Anticipated Problems	P = Treatment Plan

ADDITIONAL NOTES

© WMA, INC 1995

SOAP NOTE

SCENE

SUBJECTIVE

S Symptoms

A Allergies
M Medications
P Past History
L Last Meal
E Events

OBJECTIVE

EXAM:

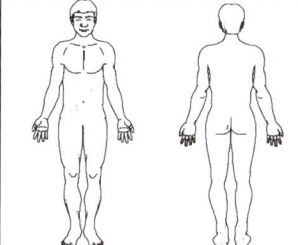

VITAL SIGNS

Time	Pulse	Resp.	B/P	Skin	Temp.	AVPU
			/			
			/			
			/			
			/			
			/			
			/			
			/			

Emergency training for outdoor professionals.™

207-665-2707 888-WILD-MED 189 Dudley Road, Bryant Pond, ME 04219 © WMA, INC 1995

ASSESSMENT AND TREATMENT PLAN

A = Assessment (Problem List)	A' = Anticipated Problems	P = Treatment Plan

ADDITIONAL NOTES

© WMA, INC 1995

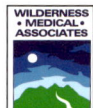

SOAP NOTE

SCENE

SUBJECTIVE

S Symptoms

A Allergies
M Medications
P Past History
L Last Meal
E Events

OBJECTIVE

EXAM:

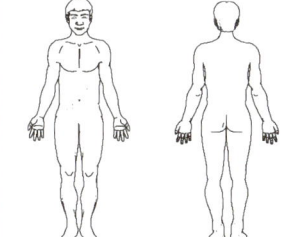

VITAL SIGNS

Time	Pulse	Resp.	B/P	Skin	Temp.	AVPU
			/			
			/			
			/			
			/			
			/			
			/			
			/			

Emergency training for outdoor professionals.™

ASSESSMENT AND TREATMENT PLAN

A = Assessment (Problem List)	A' = Anticipated Problems	P = Treatment Plan

ADDITIONAL NOTES

© WMA, INC 1996

SOAP NOTE

SCENE

SUBJECTIVE

S Symptoms

A Allergies
M Medications
P Past History
L Last Meal
E Events

OBJECTIVE

EXAM:

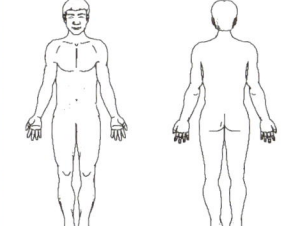

VITAL SIGNS

Time	Pulse	Resp.	B/P	Skin	Temp.	AVPU
			/			
			/			
			/			
			/			
			/			
			/			
			/			

Emergency training for outdoor professionals.™

207-665-2707 888-WILD-MED 189 Dudley Road, Bryant Pond, ME 04219 © WMA, INC 1995

ASSESSMENT AND TREATMENT PLAN

A = Assessment (Problem List)	A' = Anticipated Problems	P = Treatment Plan

ADDITIONAL NOTES

© WMA, INC 1995

Component	Examples	Evaluation	Treatment
UPPER AIRWAY (obstruction)	Cork - food Kink - Flexed Fluid - Blood Swelling - Burns	See Initial Assessment Inadequate/no air in/out Decreasing AVPU, cyanotic Survey scene for info Identify cause if possible	Attempt ventilation(PPV) Reposition airway (TIP) "POP" cork (abdominal thrusts) gravity, suction, ALS, ASAP
LOWER AIRWAY (swelling, spasm)	Anaphylaxis Asthma Irritants Infection	Respiratory Distress, Anxious Vital signs elevated Wheezes, lung sounds Pt. often has history Use PAS to find cause	**P**osition of Comfort **R**eassurance **O**2 - 100% if available **P**ositive Pressure Ventilations Medication- Bronchodialator,ALS
ALVEOLI (fluid)	Drowning CHF Smoke Inhalation HAPE Infection	Respiratory Distress Productive cough Rales, crackles Elevated vital signs	- P.R.O.P. - Medications - ALS as needed - If at altitude, descend
CHEST WALL (trauma blunt/ penetrating)	- Moderate or severe MOI - Flail chest - Open chest wound	LOOK (inspection) LISTEN (auscultation) FEEL (palpation) Respiratory distress Possible volume shock	- P.R.O.P. - ALS ASAP - Plug holes - Support injured area
NEURO DRIVE (loss of drive)	**S** - Sugar↑ **T** - Temperature↑ or ↓ **O** - Oxygen↓ **P** - Pressure **E** - Electricity **A** - Altitude **T** - Toxins **S** - Salts	Decreasing AVPU Depressed vital signs Cyanosis Possible vomiting, seizures Survey scene, use PAS to identify cause	- P.R.O.P. - ALS ASAP - Treat cause if possible - Change environment

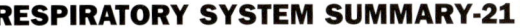

RESPIRATORY SYSTEM SUMMARY-21

(also see Asthma, pg 60-61; Respiratory Infections, pg 69-70)

CIRCULATORY SYSTEM SUMMARY-22

Component	Mechanism	Evaluation	Treatment

VOLUME SHOCK	**Volume Loss** Fast / Slow Internal / External Blood / Fluids	USE *PAS* TO DETERMINE CAUSE
		     EARLY **LATE**
		 P-elevated higher
		 R-elevated elevated
		 B/P-normal down
		 S- clammy same
		 C-anxious V,P,U
		 OTHER urine output ↓
			- Stop Loss
			 - Oral / IV Volume
			 - ALS ASAP
			 - P.R.O.P.
			   (See BLS)

CARDIO-GENIC SHOCK	**Pump Problem** CHF, MI Trauma	Pt. often has cardiac Hx P- elevated or down R- often up, labored S - clammy B/P - down	- P.R.O.P. - ALS ASAP
VASCULAR SHOCK	Anaphylaxis (p.62) Spine Injury (p.35,81-88) Sepsis	P - often elevated R - normal or elevated B/P - down S - often flushed / warm T - up if infection present	- P.R.O.P. - Medications - ALS ASAP - Spine if M.O.I.
ASR (NOT SHOCK) Acute Stress Reaction Sympathetic / Parasympathetic	**STRESS** -Speed up (rush) -Slow down (faint)	SYMPATHETIC PARASYM P - elevated down R - elevated down B/P - elevated down S - clammy clammy T - N N C - anxious temp LOC	- TIME - Reassurance - Treat other prob. *NOTE: ASR can occur with Shock*

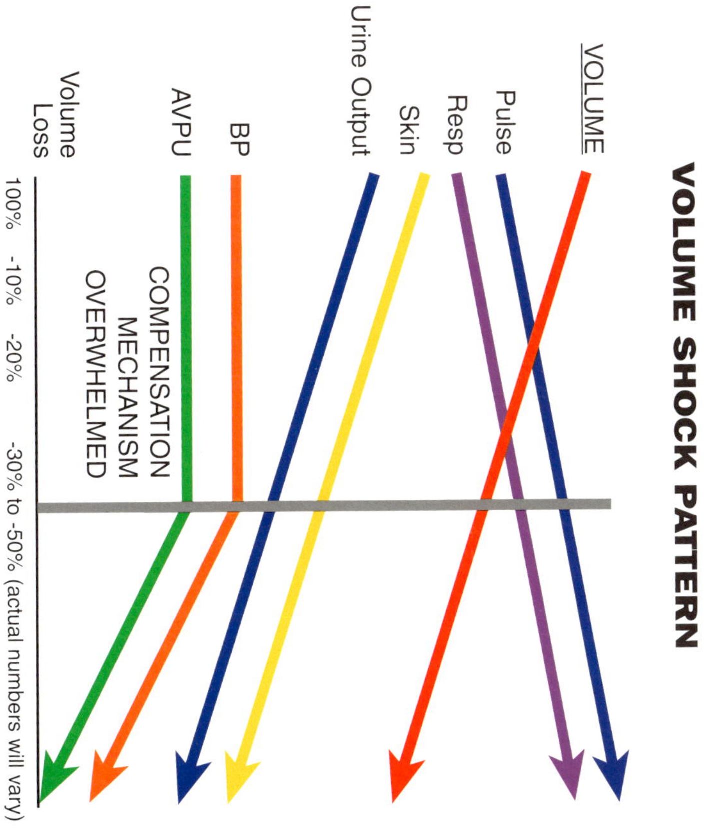

VOLUME SHOCK PATTERN

Volume Loss							VOLUME
	AVPU	BP	Urine Output	Skin	Resp	Pulse	

- 100%
- -10%
- -20%

COMPENSATION MECHANISM OVERWHELMED

- -30%
- to -50% (actual numbers will vary)

VOLUME SHOCK PATTERN-23
(also see Chest Pain, pg 63; Anaphylaxis, pg 62)

BRAIN/NERVOUS SYSTEM SUMMARY-24

(also see *Spine Injury*, pg 35-37)

Problem	Evaluation, Other Info	Treatment
CONCUSSION Trauma to Head resulting in a change of mental status - temporary loss of consciousness, amnesia	- Consider MOI → Spine injury - Use Spine assessment to rule in / out - Variable levels of amnesia - Unconscious >5 minutes, considered serious - Patient has potential to develop increasing ICP within 24 hours NOTE: If no concussion has occurred, evacuation may not be necessary	- Protect airway and spine during initial assessment - Patient should be monitored for 24 hours, evacuation should be considered - Acetaminophen okay for headache - Observe for S/Sx of ↑ICP: AVPU, headache, vomiting
INCREASING INTRACRANIAL PRESSURE (↑ICP) - severe head injury - Stroke (CVA) - High Altitude Cerebral Edema (HACE) - Other	*EARLY* Mental status changes ↓ Persistent vomiting Severe headache P - normal R - normal B/P - normal *LATE* AVPU Seizure "Blown" pupil P - down R - down B/P - up	**P**osition (spine?, vomiting?, elevate head) **R**eassurance (can't hurt) **O**2 - 100% **P**ositive pressure ventilations as needed Medications - ALS ASAP
SEIZURES - Epilepsy Hx - S.T.O.P.E.A.T.S. (See page 21)	- Aura (Patient feels seizure coming) - Decreasing AVPU (temporary) - Tonic / clonic (active seizure) - possible incontinence - post ictal state (groggy post seizure) - possibly confused	- Protect Patient - NO invasive airway tools - Evaluate for injuries - Use Patient to develop Tx/ evacuation plan - Medications - ALS ASAP for <u>multiple</u> seizures

Evaluation Criteria
Musculoskeletal Injuries
(Guidelines Only)

Mechanism of Injury	STABLE, MINOR / USUALLY MINOR	MODERATE / VARIABLE	UNSTABLE / OFTEN SEVERE
Pop, snap, crack	usually none	sometimes yes	often yes
Swelling	slow onset (6-24 H)	yes	yes
Pain, tenderness	some (variable)	yes	yes, often severe
Use after injury	limited, but yes	possible	usually none
Range of motion	full-okay	limited	limited-none
Distal C.S.M.	full-okay	usually okay	? diminished
Weight bearing ability	near normal	limited	none
"normal use"			
Deformity/angulation	no	sometimes	often yes
Feels unstable to pt.	no	sometimes	often yes
TREATMENT	- usually okay to stay in the field - RICE, PFA, Meds - ? Tape - Reevaluate	- possible evacuation, especially if in an institutional setting (client, student, etc.) - RICE, MEDS, splint?	- Treat as a fracture or unstable - Immobilize - RICE, Meds - Monitor

R est
I ce
C ompression
E levation

P ain
F ree
A ctivity

MUSCULOSKELETAL INJURY EVAL. -25

INJURY EVALUATION
SIGNS/SYMPTOMS

STABLE — **UNSTABLE**

NONSPECIFIC SIGNS/SYMPTOMS
- pain
- swelling
- tenderness
- bruising/discoloration
- pop/snap
- open/closed

SPECIFIC SIGNS/SYMPTOMS FOR UNSTABLE INJURIES
- deformity/angulation
- crepitus
- feeling of instability
- weight bearing ability
- impaired CSM

FIELD MANAGEMENT

GENERAL PRINCIPLES OF SPLINTING

- Long bone fractures should be splinted in anatomic position. Use traction into position to accomplish this.
- Stop T.I.P. if: 1) increase in pain; 2) resistance is met.
- For long bone fractures, immobilize the joint above and below.
- For joint injuries, immobilize the bone above and below.
- Joint fractures and/or dislocations are generally splinted in their presenting position unless there is a compromise in the distal circulation, sensation, motor (CSM)
- Splints should be **well-padded**, light, adjustable and multi-directional (sandwich + resist movement).
- Monitor CSM before and after splinting.
- Be prepared to adjust the splint.

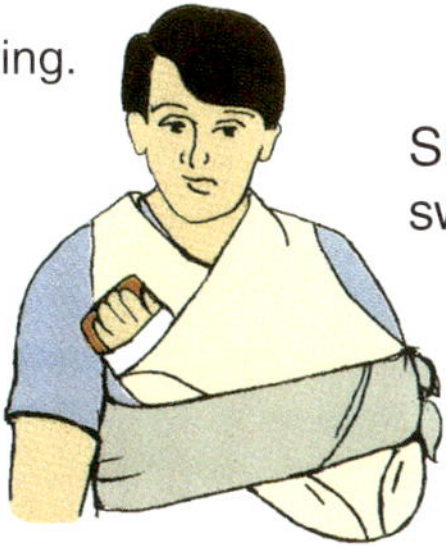

Forearm / wrist splint

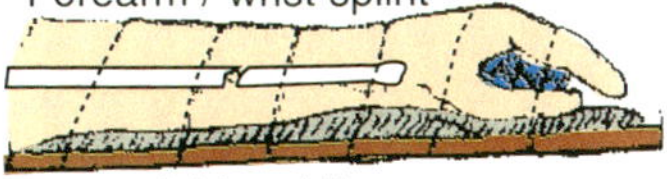

rigid padding

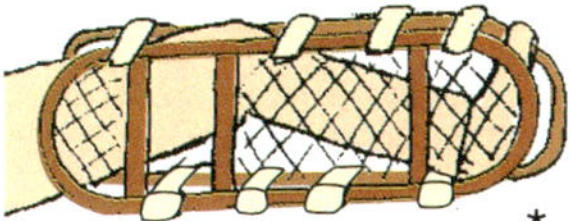

Sling and swathe

Snow shoe splint*

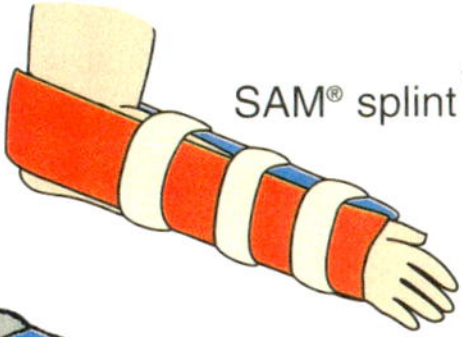

SAM® splint*

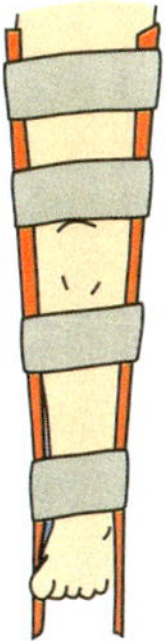

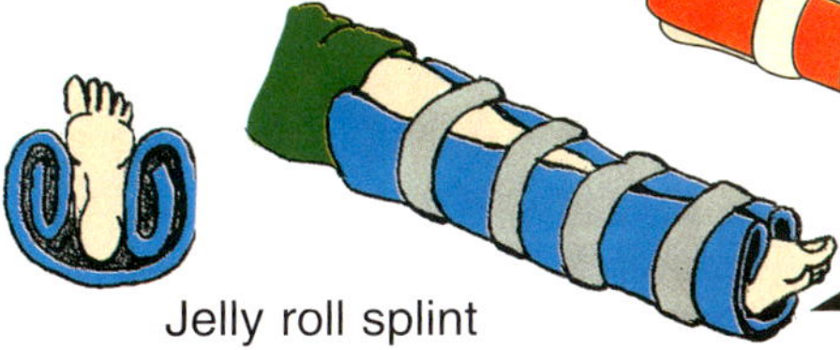

Jelly roll splint

Ensolite®

* Padding excluded in illustration for visual clarity.

MUSCULOSKELETAL SYS/SPLINTING-27
(also see pg 28-38)

MUSCULOSKELETAL/DISLOCATIONS-28

EVALUATION AND TREATMENT OF DISLOCATIONS

SEVERE DEFORMITY OR DISTAL CSM COMPROMISE?

NO

Splint in position found, monitor & evacuate

YES

Reposition towards anatomic position unless:
1) there is a significant increase in pain or;
2) physical resistance is met.

OR

IF the rescuer is :
1) trained in reduction of dislocations;
2) certified/authorized;
3) has permission from the patient and;
4) is in the prolonged/delayed transport environment.

Attempt to Reduce Dislocation in the Field.

Dislocations worthy of field reductions are:
    PATELLA: 1) Sit patient up, flex at hip.
                 2) Straighten leg.
                 3) Push medially & pop in place.
                    Post reduction, most patients can walk out.
    FINGERS & TOES: 1) Hold distal to joint.
                         2) Use traction into position.

SHOULDER:
- Patients often have prior history.
- They have limited range of motion.
- Mechanism is typically lever action where humeral head pops anterior.
- Check distal CSM before/after.

STEP 1
- Calm and reassure patient (and yourself).
- Explain the process to the patient.
- Have patient recline or lay flat.
- Pull firmly, but with gentle and smooth traction on the upper arm in the direction it is pointing.

Note deformity

STEP 2
- While maintaining traction, bring the arm out, away from the body (abduction).
- This process may take a few minutes; be patient.

STOP TIP if: Pain increases OR physical resistance is met (but don't let go).

STEP 3
- While maintaining traction, externally rotate the arm (like preparing to throw a ball). Again, be patient, this should do it.

STEP 4
- Sling and swathe.
- Consider evacuation.
- Pain and swelling will develop.

MUSCULOSKELETAL/DISLOCATIONS-29

EVALUATION / TREATMENT

DISLOCATION EVALUATION

- **WILDERNESS CONTEXT?** — NO
  - YES →
- **SHOULDER, PATELLA, DIGITS?** — NO
  - YES →
- **INDIRECT FORCE?** — NO
  - YES → **REDUCE**
- **CSM COMPROMISED?**
  - YES → **TIP** → **MANAGE AS UNSTABLE JOINT**
  - NO → **MANAGE AS UNSTABLE JOINT**

DISLOCATION EVALUATION-30

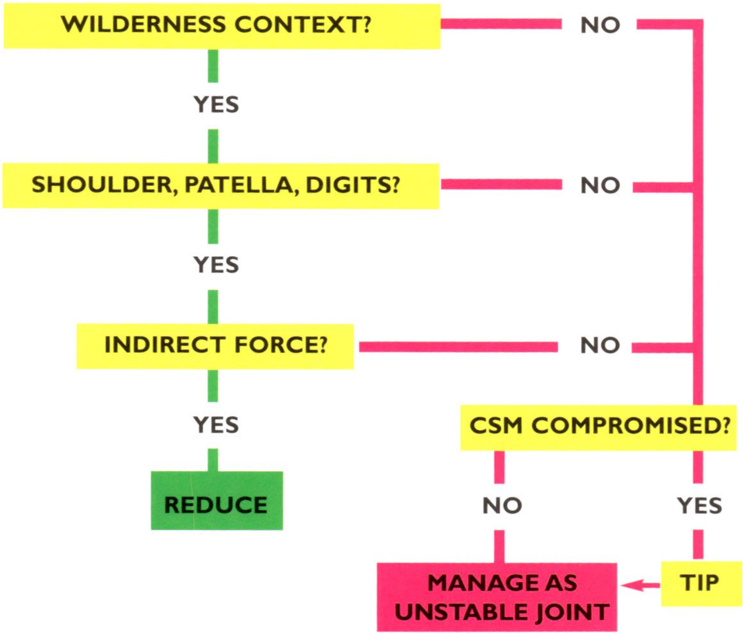

KNEES

Knee injuries can be broken down into overuse syndromes, direct trauma, twists and strains. Overuse syndrome happens when repetitive motion (cycling) or pounding (hiking downhill) causes irritation and inflammation in and around the knee. This is a usually a stable injury with the knee becoming painful and swollen. This can be treated with rest, ice, compression and elevation (RICE) and antiinflammatory meds. Traumatic injuries such as slamming a knee into a rock can be painful initially and over time degree of severity is usually apparent. The twisting, popping, and torquing mechanisms to the knee can sometimes be difficult to assess. In addition to the standard musculoskeletal assessment guidelines, the following questions and exam techniques may be of benefit:
• Was the person able to get up unassisted after the initial injury?
• Were they able to continue the activity?
• Did they hear a pop, or feel a snap in their knee? (Half the time that indicates an ACL tear)
• Did the joint swell, and if so how quickly?
• Did the knee lock up at all?

The history and physical exam of the knee are designed to help you and the patient determine the severity of the injury. You do not have an MRI or an orthopedic consult in the field, so be conservative. Many times in the field, a stable injury can be made more comfortable by bracing the injury until a more professional assessment can be obtained.

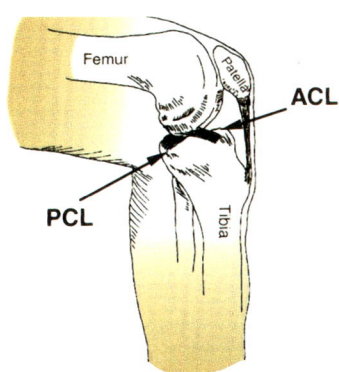

ACL - Anterior Cruciate Ligament

PCL - Posterior Cruciate Ligament

MCL - Medial Collateral Ligament

LCL - Lateral Collateral Ligament

MUSCULOSKELETAL INJURY EVAL. - 32

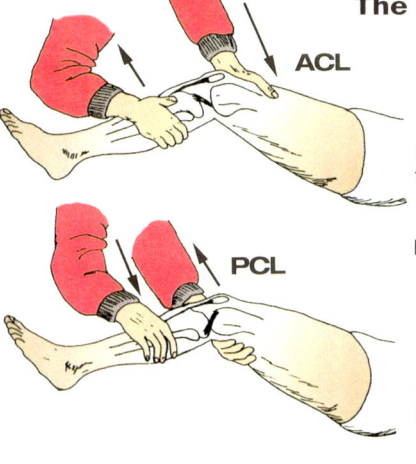

The Cruciate Ligament Test

This will help determine the stability of the ACL and PCL.

To check the ACL, stabilize the distal thigh, and reach behind the tibial plateau, and pull the proximal tib-fib anteriorly to "draw" the tib-fib forward. If the area draws out and creates a shelf-like appearance, this may indicate an ACL tear. This may not be painful if the ligament is torn, as there are no stretch receptors to register the pain.

To check the PCL, the leg should be flexed 15-20°, hold under the distal thigh, just above the knee with one hand, and push the proximal tibial plateau posteriorly with the other hand. Note: normal findings (negative) should not cause pain, and there should be a solid end point, not mushy, or boggy.

Collateral Ligament Test

The collateral ligaments are tested by anchoring the knee on one side at a time, and then levering the lower leg to stress the collateral ligaments. Again, normal findings should elicit no tenderness, and should find a "solid" end point.

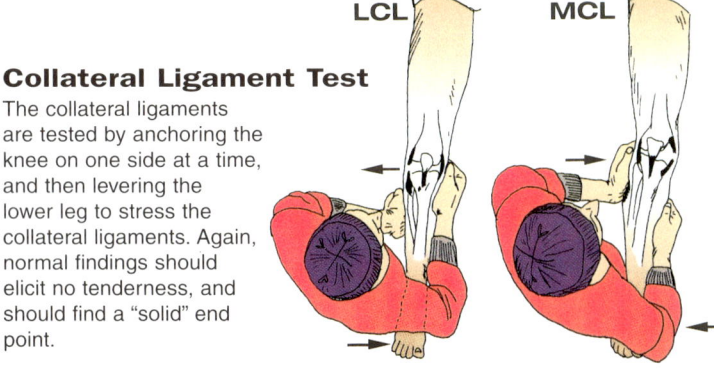

ANKLE INJURIES

Ankle injuries are the most common musculoskeletal injury encountered in the wilderness. Improper footwear, being poorly conditioned, and prior history of ankle problems increase the risk of injury. A careful look at the MOI, exam findings, weight bearing ability, and history will help to determine the appropriate course of action. Not all ankle injuries need to be evacuated for radiographic studies (x-rays).

Most ankle injuries are from inversion (rotating/twisting the ankle inward).

ANKLE EXAMINATION

Go through the standard evaluation for musculoskeletal injuries. If you are in doubt about the need for evacuation for x-rays for a person with an ankle injury, try this more detailed evaluation. Often referred to as the Ottawa Ankle Rules, this test is used in many EDs to determine whether or not to order an x-ray. A completely normal exam means that a fracture of the ankle and forefoot is highly unlikely. If abnormalities are noted the urgency of the evacuation can be determined on a case by case basis.

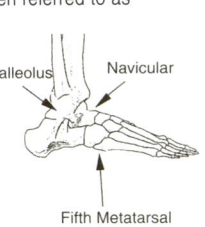

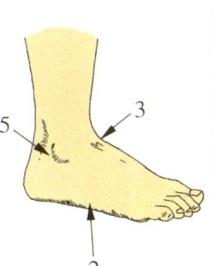

This specific ankle evaluation has 5 components that must all be present in order to be reasonably certain that there are no fractures:

- 1. The patient must be able to bear weight on the injured foot without significant pain. This must be true initially after the traumatic event and also during the evaluation (which might be done later).
- 2. No point tenderness to the base of the fifth metatarsal.
- 3. No point tenderness to the navicular bone.
- 4. No point tenderness to the posterior edge or tip of the medial malleolus.
- 5. No point tenderness to the posterior edge or tip of the lateral malleolus.

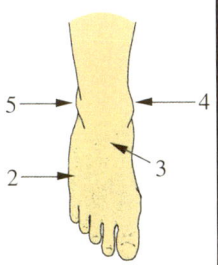

If all of these findings are negative, then it is highly unlikely that there is any fracture.

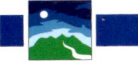

MUSCULOSKELETAL INJURY EVAL. - 33

MUSCULOSKELETAL INJURY EVAL. - 34

MANAGEMENT OF ANKLE INJURIES

If evacuation is indicated, the patient may be able to walk out with a weight bearing splint/brace using a SAM™ splint or a good taping job. Taping and/or bracing can also be used to stabilize an ankle injury, allowing the person to remain on the trip.

USING TAPE TO STABILIZE AN ANKLE

• Taping an ankle is best done after the swelling goes down. Try to avoid circumferential (all the way around) taping. 2" athletic tape works well.

• Do not use duct tape if at all possible (it was never meant to go on human skin, and it does not breathe.)

• Start with clean, dry feet.

• Start taping under the foot on the arch side, then smoothly come up and around the injured area, and wrap around the ankle, 2 or 3 strips should be enough.

• Use longer tape lengths to make strips from mid-calf on one side of the leg, under the heel area, and up the other side to mid-calf (again, 2-3 strips should work well).

• Taping is usually only good for one day at a time.

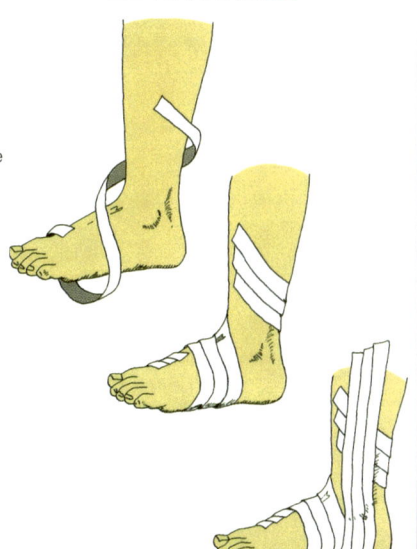

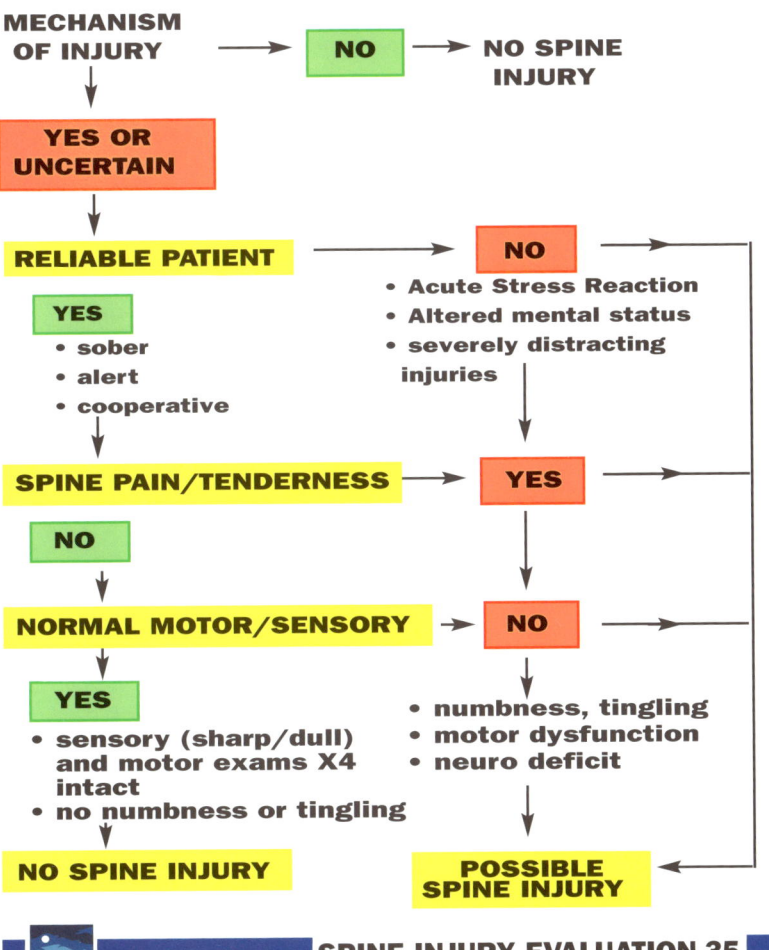

NERVOUS/SPINE INJURY CARE-36

GENERAL RULES

• If spine injury cannot be ruled out, then patient should be immobilized fully and evacuated.

• The spine-injured patient is best immobilized on a backboard, vacuum mattress or rigid litter.

• Apply a cervical collar on the patient as soon as can be done safely (manufactured or improvised).

• Remember that a collar alone does not immobilize the spine.

• Movement of the patient should be directed at bringing them back into anatomic position unless increased pain or resistance is met.

• Axial movement of the patient is usually easier and safer than side-ways movement. The rescuer on the head should call movement of the patient. She/he should use clear, simple command: "Ready to lift . . . lift." Do not pull head.

• Movement should be done in small increments.

• If you must leave the patient to get help, he/she may be better off on their side to better protect the airway.

• Significant padding is indicated under and around the patient; also under the knees, buttocks, heels and the back of the head.

• If the patient is awake and cooperative, there is no need to tie their hands together.

• The patient can be moved bare-handed short distances to better protect them from the environment. Training and practice is required.

• Remember, some cord injured patients developed their injuries *after* their initial insult!

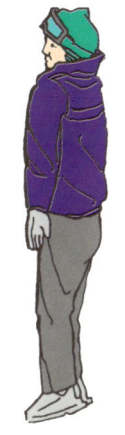
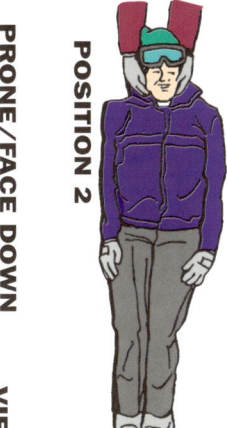
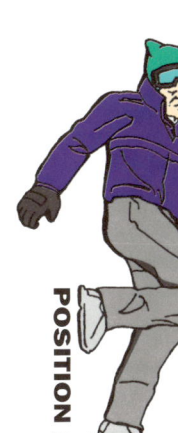
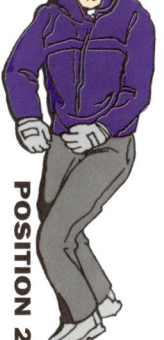

NERVOUS/BASIC BODY POSITIONS-37
(also see Spine Injury Management, pg 81-82; and Improvised Spine Immobilization and Litters, pg 83-88)

MUSCULOSKEL/FRACTURED FEMUR-38

FRACTURES OF THE FEMUR AND PELVIS

Fractured femurs deserve particular attention because they are very painful and can lead to significant blood loss. The powerful spasms of the thigh muscles cause further tissue damage.

• There is usually a significant MOI to cause one of these fractures, so use the spine assessment guidelines to rule in/out a possible spine injury. Use the PAS to determine if there are other injuries.

• The injured leg is often shortened, swollen, and the foot rotated externally. Distal CSM may be impaired.

• There can be bruising around the pelvis. The pelvis may feel unstable and there may be a significant increase in pain with any movement.

• **SPLINTING – Femur:** Traction splints are used for stabilization and support of an open or closed fractured femur. They can often releive some pain and help prevent further tissue damage. However, most manufactured splints are not convenient to carry in the backcountry. When placed on a patient, they oftentimes stick out beyond a litter and will not fit into many evacuation helicopters. The KDT-type is an exception. Improvised splints are unsatisfactory for a variety of reason. With few exceptions (e.g. Sager®), it is difficult to gauge and maintain a steady and safe tension. CSM problems can occur if left on for more than 2 hours, especially if unconscious or if frostbite is possible. **If used, monitor carefully and regularly.** A well padded buddy splint and a proper litter packing job, especially with a full body vacuum splint, provide a good alternative.

Pelvis: Pelvic stabilization with circumferential binding can help to control pain and limit bleeding. A binding device can be improvised with a rain fly or waist strap of a back pack, for example. Apply them so that the pressure is focused over the greater trochanters of the femur. Tighten enough to stabilize and for comfort. Make sure that the binder is smooth and well padded. Remove items from pockets and plan for the effects of zippers, buttons, or other hard objects that could be compressed into the skin by the binder. Monitor regularly. As with a fractured femur, proper litter packaging is essential.

• Involve ALS early for volume replacement and pain control.

NOTES

WOUNDS/IMPALED OBJECTS-40

SEVERE BLEEDING

- *Survey scene, gloves on.*
- *Expose area, visualize wound.*
- *Well-aimed direct pressure.*
- *Pressure dressing (compression wrap over dressing).*
- *Evacuate as needed.*

MINOR, MODERATE WOUNDS

- *Stop bleeding.*
- *Clean wound to minimize infection:*
  - wash skin around wound with soap & water
  - irrigate wound with water under pressure
  - pick out foreign material
- *If wound is high risk, ADD:*
  - dilute povidone iodine 1% to irrigate wound
  - consider antibiotics Rx
  - evaluate tetanus status (evacuate within 24 hour if tetanus is outdated: 10 years for clean wound;<5 years for high risk/dirty).
- *Consider rabies when animal bites are:*
  - 1) Unprovoked; 2) high risk species; 3) if animal's behavior is abnormal.

IMPALED OBJECTS

Removal of some impaled objects might make sense when in a wilderness or delayed transport situation if:
  - It is simple and easy to remove.
  - If it cannot be safely stabilized in place.
  - It would prevent safe packaging and transport.

NOTE: Authorization may be required in some situations, such as a wilderness EMS rescue team.

BURN EVALUATION

EVALUATION - SYSTEMS ORIENTED

RESPIRATORY: Inhalation injury
CIRCULATORY: Volume loss
NERVOUS: ASR / Pain
  ↓ mental status / ↓ AVPU

SKIN: Infection / Hypothermia

BURN TREATMENT

TREATMENT: SPECIFIC TO SYSTEMS INVOLVED

BURN CARE

- Stop burning (cool H2O)
- Pain medications

- **CHEMICAL BURNS**
- Stop burning: wet & dry indications
- Pain medications

- **CLEAN** - Sterile H2O, 0.5% PI
- Debridement
- Antibiotic ointments (<1% TBSA only)

- Dress - non-stick gauze
- Elevate

MINOR BURNS
Monitor for infection

MAJOR BURNS
EVACUATE
ALS / Burn center

WOUNDS/IMPALED OBJECTS-41

BLISTER CARE-42

BLISTER CARE

- Most blisters can be avoided with proper footwear and some preventive measures.
- A snug fitting liner sock or Neosocks® under a second layer of wool or polypropylene sock works well.
- Use Spenco Adhesive Knit® or Moleskin® on blister prone areas prior to an excursion. This can be applied as a simple covering. Tincture of Benzoin will help toughen the skin and help with adhesion of the tape. People may have good results using duct tape. Clean the skin with alcohol first.

HOT SPOTS

- Hot spots are the red, painful areas of irritation and friction before they become a true blister. This is a stop and fix situation, as they are relatively easy to treat at this point.
- Hot spots can be effectively treated with bandage-type covering made from tape, Moleskin or Adhesive Knit. Cut a piece of the material a bit bigger than the hot spot. This will be the "dressing" part of the bandage. Put dressing over the blister and cover with Moleskin or Adhesive Knit This can then be placed over the affected area. This works like a bandaid, but it holds better and lasts longer.

BLISTERS

- A fluid filled blister is best treated by leaving the blister intact. If you are planning to continue on your trip however, then it may make more sense to drain and clean it under clean conditions. Clean the area around the blister and using a clean needle, drain the fluid from the blister. Next, apply an antibiotic ointment like neosporin or a water-gel dressing like Spenco Second Skin®. Then cover the area using the same technique for hot spots. A second technique involves making a doughnut-type cover that keeps pressure off the drained blister. Molefoam® works well for this.

NOTES

HYPOTHERMIA-44

HYPOTHERMIA

Hypothermia occurs when the cold challenge (cold, wind, wet) over-whelms the body's ability to produce and retain heat. The following can happen: 1. Acute or immersion (minutes-hours) cold water exposure.

2. Sub-acute (hours-days) usually outdoor activities.

3. Chronic (days-weeks) elderly, babies, ill.

All of these types can be mild, moderate or severe. General hypother-mia Tx: 1) minimizing or reversing the cold challenge; 2) increasing heat production; and 3) increasing heat retention.

MILD/MODERATE HYPOTHERMIA
(96°-90° F, 35.5°-32° C)

EVALUATION
- mental status changes
- lethargic
- irritable
- withdrawn
- shivering (usually persistent)

- loss of fine motor coordination
- shell → core shunt

TREATMENT
- general Tx (above)
- reverse cold challenge
- increase heat retention (insulate)
- increase calories, hydration
- increase heat production (exercise after food, fluids admin. and mental status improves)
- treat other problems
  - evacuate?

SEVERE HYPOTHERMIA (BELOW 90° F, 32° C)
EVALUATION
- severe ↑ in mental status, then decreasing AVPU
- no shivering
- metabolic icebox
- decreased pulse
- decreased resp.
- decreased B/P

TREATMENT
- treat gently (prevent V-fib.)
- add heat packs to thorax
- minimize cold challenge
- remove cold, wet layers & insulate
- no aggressive shell rewarming (i.e., no hot tub immersion)
- evacuate to controlled rewarming. Call ALS.

ALS
- heated humidified 02 PPV
  - heated IV fluids
  - drugs: glucose, narcan, ACLS ↑ 86°F, 30°C

HYPOTHERMIA PACKAGING

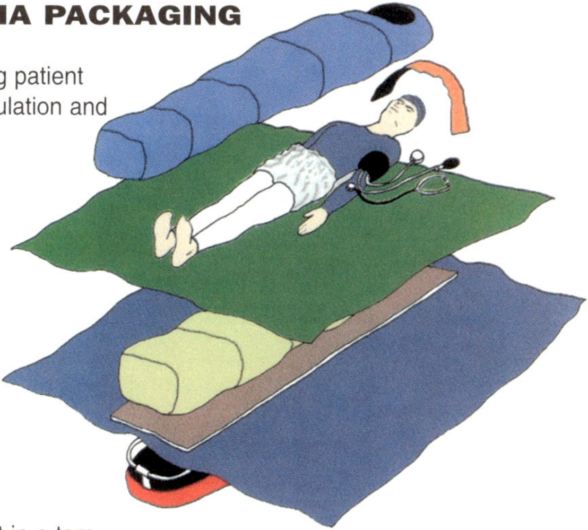

• Start by sandwiching patient between layers of insulation and waterproof layers.

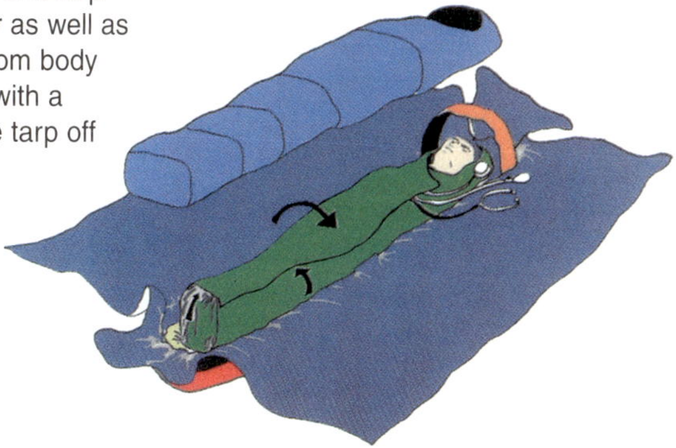

• Wrapping the patient in a tarp creates a vapor barrier as well as protecting insulation from body fluids. Making a hoop with a SAM™ splint keeps the tarp off the patient's face.

HYPOTHERMIA-46

HYPOTHERMIA PACKAGING, CONT.

• Fold ends in over patient, then fold corners as shown

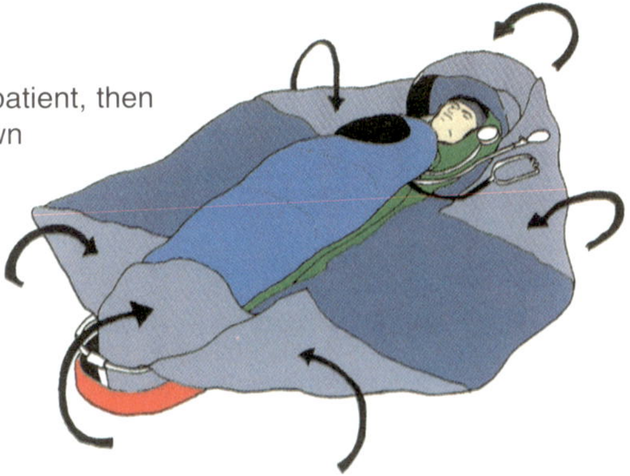

• Fold sides over, keeping wrinkles to a minimum (no wrinkles help to shed water and snow)

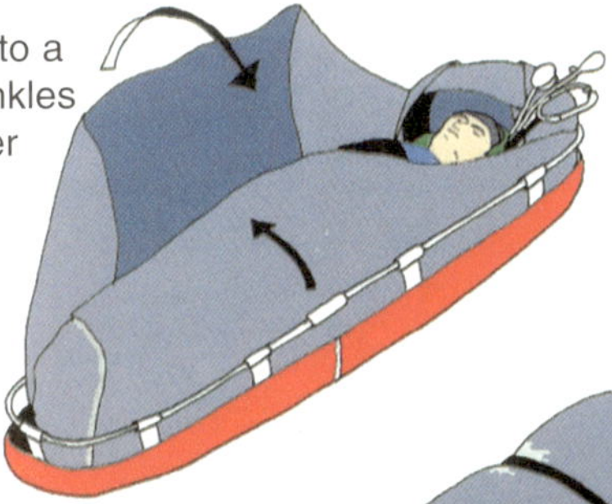

• Strap the hypo wrap package snugly in place

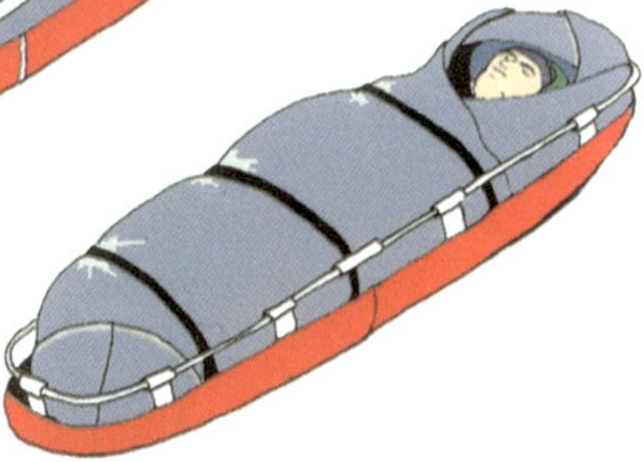

FROSTBITE

Frostbite is the actual freezing of the water in the cells. Areas most prone are extremities (ear lobes, nose, fingers, toes). Contributing factors include hypothermia, prior cold injury, dehydration, exhaustion, constriction (tight boots, straps), vasoconstrictors (caffeine, nicotine) and exposure to cold, wind (cheeks, nose).

Field Findings Before Rewarming	Treatment	Post Rewarming Results & Guidelines
cold, discomfort: exam-cold, soft (CSM-normal) **PARTIAL THICKNESS FROSTBITE** *numbness* exam-pale and hard; (CSM reduced)	• field rewarming (skin to skin, heat packs, warm H20) • general rewarming • loosen constrictive clothing/straps • rewarming is painful; use powerful pain meds if available • maintain calorie/H20 intake	• Generally there are no blisters, therefore minimal tissue damage • this result is considered superficial • prevent reoccurrence • okay to stay in the field
FULL THICKNESS FROSTBITE *numbness* exam-pale and hard; possible ice crystals (CSM absent)	• *in most circumstances evacuate to controlled rewarming* (i.e., It's ok to walk out on frozen feet) • serious pain medicine • 30 minute immersion of frozen area in 105° H20 • dry, sterile dressings **IMPORTANT :** *Post rewarming* • no use of area • no refreezing	*Post rewarming results:* **BLISTERS?** NO / YES → clear=2° bloody=3° dark, perfusion=4° • protect area • prevent use of affected areas • prevent refreezing

HEAT PROBLEMS-48

HEAT-RELATED PROBLEMS

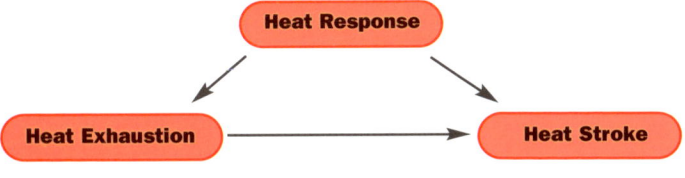

- Heat stroke is one of the leading killers of athletes in the world. Train and acclimatize to the heat. This will take about 3 weeks to do. Stay well hydrated; you may even have to back off a little when it's very hot out.

- Sweat losses in humans can easily exceed 2 liters per hour during moderate exercise in hot environments. So, take at least 1 liter an hour to help to offset the losses. You must take in some foods to replace the electrolyte losses as well. Rest and rehydration breaks are critical as humans can only absorb about 1 liter/hour.

- Certain medicines/drugs may predispose individuals to heat-related emergencies. These include psychotropics, alcohol, stimulants, antihistamines, decongestants, ephedrine, diuretics, some drugs used to control blood pressure and heart rate or rhythm.

- Cardiovascular and respiratory emergency calls (chest pain, shortness of breath) increase by about 10 fold during heat waves.

- It is estimated that 1 out of 10 cases of heat related illness are actually hyponatremia, a condition where sodium (and possibly other electrolyte) levels have been depleted through sweat losses without proper replacement. SO: Take in electrolytes as well as fluids. This can be done with "power drinks" or simply with food. Just about any foods will give you the electrolytes that you need. Frequent munching on small amounts is a good technique.

- Heat stroke may or may not be preceded by heat exhaustion. Those who are heat exhausted are dehydrated, and if they continue working in a hot environment, heat stroke may follow. A hydrated individual may develop heat stroke without ever being dehydrated. Exercise in a hot environment can cause heat stroke very quickly.

HEAT PROBLEMS

PROBLEMS	CAUSE(S)	EVALUATION	TREATMENT
Heat Exhaustion	• Fluid losses (sweat) exceeding fluid intake • Often during exercise in hot, humid environments • Most common in unacclimatized, dehydrated persons NOTE: sweat losses can exceed 2.5 liters per hour • Electrolyte losses are common	• Pulse - often elevated • Respirations - normal or elevated • B/P - normal or decreased (postural vital sign changes often noticed) • Temp - normal or slightly elevated • AVPU - awake • Signs/symptoms-dizzy, nausea, vomiting, headache, chills, often feels lightheaded • low water intake, low electrolyte intake • low urine output	• Stop exercise • Rehydrate • Replace electrolytes • Rest in a cool environment • Evacuation may not be necessary, however, make attempts to prevent recurrence
Heat Stroke Risk factors: • unfit • obese • cardiac Hx • elderly • athletes who are working hard in hot temps	• Severe, life-threatening rise in body temperature which may or may not be preceded by heat exhaustion. The body is producing more heat than it can "dump" through evaporation and other cooling mechanisms.	• Severely altered mental status followed by decreasing AVPU • Seizures are common • Pulse - elevated • Respirations - elevated • B/P - often decreased • Skin - 50% of victims are sweating, 50% are dry • Temp - above 105º F (40.5ºC)	• Radical cooling! cool water immersion or evaporative cooling technique (wet pt & fan aggressively) • IV volume replacement • ALS evacuation *Heat stroke victims often have permanent problems after recovery.*
Hyponatremia	• Excessive water intake • Low electrolyte intake Basically, the problem is that the person is sweating out lots of water and electrolytes (salts), replacing only water. This causes severe electrolyte depletion over time.	• Dizziness, nausea, vomiting, headache, chills, possible ataxia (inability to walk a straight line) • Pulse - often normal • Respirations - variable • B/P - normal or slightly elevated • Skin - normal to cool • Temp. - normal to slightly decreased • AVPU - variable • Near normal to increased urination	Abnormal mental status or significant neurological S/Sx NO → sit it out, wait it out, pee it out YES → ALS evacuation ASAP

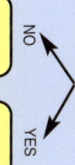

HEAT PROBLEMS-49

DROWNING / NEAR-DROWNING

- Estimated about 8,000 deaths a year in the U.S.A. Most are males; alcohol involved in many cases.
- Drowning is second leading cause of death in people under 25 years of age.
- Consider other problems (trauma, hypothermia, medical, scuba, drugs, etc.).
- Salt water is twice as lethal as fresh because of impurities. Treatment, however, is the same for both. Water cannot be effectively "drained" from the lungs.

Prevention = Education - Adult supervision will minimize risks and injuries.
- Always wear a properly fitted life jacket; use helmets when appropriate.
- Learn to swim; stay away from intoxicants; buddy up.

Rescue: Rescuer safety is paramount. REACH , THROW, ROW + GO rule applies. Avoid becoming the second victim.

Category	Evaluation/Assessment	Treatment
I. MINOR	Awake/alert during entire event. Pt may have swallowed and/or aspirated a small amount of water; possible some coughing noted. Usually a self-rescue. Healthy individuals are usually okay.	• check for injuries • evacuation optional • if pt has significant PMH, consider evacuation
II. SERIOUS	Awake, but often totally exhausted. Usually has to be rescued. Pt. has probably swallowed and/or aspirated water and may present with vomiting, respiratory distress, cough. Potential to develop respiratory problems, particularly if LOC.	• evaluate for other injuries • evacuation • consider ALS intercept • O2, general respiratory Tx
III. CRITICAL	Often prolonged exposure, submersion. May be in respiratory failure/arrest, or cardiac arrest. Consider other problems; hypothermia, trauma, etc. If scuba is involved, call DAN 919/684-8111 and consider helicopter evacuation to decompression chamber.	• BLS/ALS ASAP • consider MOI (spine) • general resp/circ Tx **P.R.O.P.** • treat other problems

SCUBA DIVING INJURIES

- There are many specific problems related to scuba diving. Two of the more serious problems are arterial gas embolus (AGE) and decompression sickness (the Bends).
- Most divers will be very knowledgeable about diving related problems.
- Use the Divers Alert Network (DAN) based out of Duke University to help make an evacuation plan. They can be reached at (919) 684-8111
- If the patient is to be flown out by helicopter, try to stay below 1000' (330m)

	Decompression Sickness (Bends)	Arterial Gas Embolus (AGE)
Mechanism	• Due to a rapid ascent that does not allow for the release of excess nitrogen accumulated in the body while breathing at a depth > 33' (10m) (nitrogen accumulation increases as depth and time under water increase) • Caused by too much nitrogen coming out of solution, back into a gas, inside the body • Often associated with repeat dives (bounce dives) or deep dives	• Due to rapid decrease in pressure (too rapid ascent) w/inadequate venting of expanding gas. (e.g. breath holding) even at swimming pool depths • Air embolism travels into the systemic circulation causing arterial blockages, ischemia, necrosis (heart, brain) • Subcutaneous air and pneumothorax can also develop
Assessment	• Onset somewhat delayed (minutes-hours) • Wide range of S/Sx including joint aches, skin rash, chest pain, respiratory distress	• Fast onset (minutes) • May present with brain and heart ischemia signs and symptoms (chest pain, shortness of breath, dizziness, one-sided or diffuse neurological deficits) • May develop these S/Sx before surfacing
Treatment		• Same general treatment for both AGE and the bends • BLS/ALS as needed, PROP • If possible, go to an ED and have them call DAN immediately after their assessment. • Arrange for evacuation to hyperbaric chamber ASAP • Transport diving equipment with patient so it can be checked out • give 100% oxygen if possible • Attempt to procure patient's dive profile

LIGHTNING-52

LIGHTNING

- No place outside is safe when thunderstorms are in the area.
- Lightning can occur without rain or visable clouds in the sky.
- Some experts believe that the real number of deaths from lightning strikes has not been accurately tallied and that the numbers may in fact be higher than those reported. We do know that not everyone who is hit dies.
- Lightning's direct current effects generally 'flashover' the outside of the body, rarely causing entrance/exit wounds.
- Acute injuries can include cardio-respiratory arrest, heart dysrhythmias, paralysis, concussion, ruptured eardrums, skin burns, and fractures. Potential for delayed problems with kidney function, eye/cataract problems, and development of PTSD (post traumatic stress disorder) warrant hospital follow-up for any lightning strike victim.
- Immediately evacuate any patient who has recovered from cardiac arrest, been struck in the head, has any neurologic injury, or sustained burn or other injury.
- Rescuers must continually assess and consider scene safety.

Category/Evaluation	Treatment
I. MINIMALLY INJURED Patient awake and alert; Shaken up. May have ruptured eardrum or minor s/sx. *NOTE:* victims don't stay "charged."	• requires observation • measured evacuation • consider other injuries
II. SERIOUSLY INJURED Often found unconscious; possible superficial burns. May have or develop cardiac, nervous, or respiratory problems.	• treat injuries as needed • evacuation • check for other injuries
III. CRITICALLY INJURED Often found in cardio-respiratory arrest which may or may not respond to treatment. Other findings might include: paralysis; cardiac dysrhythmias; respiratory failure; decreased AVPU.	• BLS/ALS ASAP • immediate ALS evacuation • if patient is in full arrest, consider stopping CPR after 30 minutes • consider other injuries

LIGHTNING PREVENTION

- Know the local weather patterns.
- Seek shelter when you hear thunder or see lightning. Lightning strikes can occur whenever the time from the lightning flash to the thunder crash is less than 30 seconds.
  Remember: Lightning can strike even when it is not raining and when there are no clouds visible in the sky.
- Avoid being in exposed areas during potential storms such as creeks, cracks, crevices, ridges, towers/high places, open water, isolated tall objects, and openings of caves or buildings.
- Spread the group out but maintain visual contact if possible. Get low; insulate from the ground current by sitting or squatting on non-conductive padding such as ensolite, ropes, or other padding.
- The storm path can be estimated by counting the seconds between lightning bolt and thunderclap and by dividing by 3 to give approximate distance in kilometers from the storm front. (miles, divide by 5) Continue to drill for up to 30 minutes after lightning last seen or heard. (30/30 rule-pg. 95)

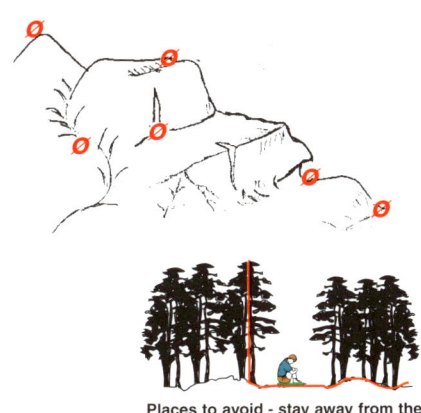

Places to avoid - stay away from the base of trees, rocks, shallow caves and overhangs.

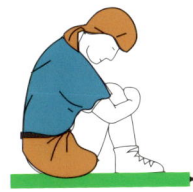

LIGHTNING POSITION

LIGHTNING-53

HIGH ALTITUDE-54

ALTITUDE SICKNESS

Altitude sickness is caused by going high faster than our bodies can acclimatize. Atmospheric pressure decreases as altitude increases; therefore, there is less available oxygen at high altitudes. The percentage of O2 remains the same (about 21%). Humans adapt to the hypoxic stress over time by hyperventilating and adjusting a myriad of processes including cardiac output, pH, red blood cell production, oxygen use, just to name a few. Most problems at altitude are preventable.

The following are guidelines:
- Train both for endurance and strength before going to high elevations.
- Maintain adequate hydration and nutrition. A high carbohydrate diet (70%) may decrease AMS (acute mountain sickness) signs/symptoms by up to 30%.
- Ascend gradually to allow for acclimatization. Above 10,000 feet (3000 meters) ascend no more than 2,000 - 3,000 feet (750 - 1000 meters) in a 24 hour period. Take a rest day every 2-3 days.
- Until acclimatized, avoid excessive exercise and fatigue. The use of certain medicines and techniques may minimize problems.

GUIDELINES FOR TREATMENT OF ACUTE MOUNTAIN SICKNESS (AMS):

1. Do not go higher with any AMS signs/symptoms; take a rest day or descend.
2. Descend if signs/symptoms do not improve within 24 hours.
3. Descend immediately with severe AMS: high altitude pulmonary edema (HAPE), high altitude cerebral edema (HACE) and do not send affected individuals down by themselves.

ACUTE MOUNTAIN SICKNESS (AMS)

Problems/Evaluation Criteria	Treatment
MILD AMS: S/Sx similar to feeling hung over: headache, nausea, insomnia, fatigue, lack of appetite; usually develops over 8000 feet (2500 meters) elevation.	• stop ascent; rest day(s) • maintain adequate hydration & nutrition • meds for pain, nausea & acclimatization
MODERATE TO SEVERE AMS: More significant or unresolved mild AMS S/Sx.	• same as above, but descent should be mandatory and immediate. • Gamow Bag® if available • emergency meds:
HIGH ALTITUDE PULMONARY EDEMA (HAPE): • shortness of breath, cough, cyanosis • rales (fluid in lungs) gurgling • respiratory + cardiac rate increasing	• general resp. Tx (PROP) • Gamow Bag® if available • emergency meds:
HIGH ALTITUDE CEREBRAL EDEMA (HACE): • mental status changes (confusion, lethargy • decreased consciousness (AVPU) • severe headache • vomiting	• general resp. Tx (PROP) • Gamow Bag® if available • emergency meds: • consider ALS intercept

Medicines for Acclimatization and Rescue:

Acetazolamide - (Diamox®) assists in acclimatization by adjusting pH. 125-250 mg. every 8-12 hours Dosages may be reduced as symptoms are resolved.

Dexamethazone - (Decadron®) a steroid to reduce edema; good for moderate - severe HACE. Available both in IM (injectable) or oral (4 mg every 6 hours) until descent to safe elevation.

Nifedipine - (Procardia®) a calcium channel blocker effective at reducing HAPE (20 mg sub-lingual, then 20 mg every 6 hours).

Sildenifil (Viagara®) - A vasodilator showing promise.

NOTE: These medicines are prescription drugs. Consult a physician and educate yourself prior to using them.

Inhaler Beta agonists (e.g. salmeterol) may help prevent HAPE.

HIGH ALTITUDE / PROBLEMS-55

TOXINS, BITES AND STINGS (General Notes)

- Toxins can produce local or systemic effects ranging from minor to critical.
- Identification of the specific toxin may be easy, or impossible, as they may be mixed/ unknown.
- The goal in treatment is to remove and dilute, if possible, and allow the body to metabolize, then excrete the toxin. Support of vital functions and lessening s/sx is appropriate. Antidotes are available for some toxins.

Toxin Type	Evaluation/Assessment	Treatment
INGESTED TOXINS:	• S/Sx range from nothing, upset stomach, to totally unresponsive, coma, or death. May involve multiple big 3 systems. Try to determine: 1) what?; 2) when?; 3) how much?	• General treatment (above) • Most authorities do not recommend syrup of Ipecac to induce vomiting. Instead use activated charcoal to bind toxin. • Evacuate
SNAKE ENVENOMATION: CROTALIDS: Rattlesnake Copperhead Cottonmouth (Water Moccasin) ELAPIDS: Coral snake	No envenomation in 20 - 30% of bites. All of these pit vipers have similar envenomation S/Sx that tend to be immediate and profound: 1) significant swelling, discoloration; and 2) significant pain at site. 3) possible systemic reaction Little-no local S/Sx. Delayed neurologic S/Sx, including numbness, headache & eventual muscular paralysis is possible.	• Remove constricting articles • Clean area, dress wound • Mark edema to determine rate and amount of swelling • Walk pt. out if he/she is able • No need to kill snake.
ARTHROPOD ENVENOMATION: stinging insects bees, wasps, fire ants	Local pain, swelling, redness, inflammation, occasionally with multiple stings. Pt. may develop malaise, nausea, vomiting, fever. Some people may develop anaphylaxis (pg 62).	• Scrape/pick off poison sac as needed. • wash/clean area • Sawyer Extractor® may help • meat tenderizer, baking soda • antihistamines for systemic reaction

TOXINS, BITES & STINGS

Toxin Type	Evaluation/Assessment	Treatment
SPIDER BITES: **Black Widow** Body - 1.0-1.5 cm Legs - 4.0-5.0 cm Venom - neurotoxic	Mild pin prick followed by severe muscle cramping and pain progressing to chest, back, abdomen and limbs. Occasionally pt. will present with hypertension, respiratory distress, paralysis, and seizures.	• oral/IV analgesics • muscle relaxants • evacuate; consider ALS • antihypertensive meds if needed
Brown Recluse Body - 1.0-1.5 cm Legs - 4.0-5.0 cm Violin shape on back Venom - local necrosis	Usually painless bite; within 6-12 hr, bull's eye lesion develops with blistering/redness that resembles a cigar burn. Area sometimes enlarges and can become necrotic. Systemic S/Sx usually minimal; can be severe.	• local wound care • ice packs may help
SCORPION STINGS: Can sting multiple times.	Most species cause significant local pain and swelling with little to no systemic effects. The centruroides species found in Arizona can present with serious systemic effects.	• cold packs • oral analgesics
MARINE TOXINS: **Nematocysts:** • jelly fish • corals • anemones	Local pain, tenderness, swelling, much like many bee stings. Minimal systemic S/Sx unless massive injection. Many unfired nematocysts may still be on victim.	• do not rub or rinse with fresh water as this will stimulate firing • saltwater rinse • soak in alcohol or vinegar • scrape off remaining sacs • apply meat tenderizer • alcohol or vinegar possibly helpful • soak in hot water; 105°F+, non-scalding, for 30 -90 min. or until pain lowered (inactivates toxin) • remove stinger as needed • generic wound care
Spiny Injuries: • sting rays • catfish	Usually one or a few puncture wounds with severe pain, and tenderness. Systemic S/Sx variable	

Toxin Type	Evaluation/Assessment	Treatment
TICK DISEASES: Lyme Disease Deer tick # 1 High risk areas: • Northeast • upper Mid-west • California • Nevada	Lyme disease is a progressive, debilitating disease transmitted by ticks. Ticks must be implanted for at least 24 hrs. to transmit bacteria to humans. **STAGE 1:** (days-weeks) - expanding red rash around site: flu-like s/sx may develop: fever, HA, fatigue, joint pains. **STAGE 2:** (weeks-months) - neurologic problems (meningitis, Bells palsy). Cardiac abnormalities infection, rashes. **STAGE 3:** (months-years) -Circulatory, respiratory, and nervous system problems, severe arthritis s/sx.	• antibiotics: doxycycline, amoxicillin • same (NOTE: early treatment is most effective • same • same
Rocky Mountain Spotted Fever: High risk areas: • Montana • Carolinas	**STAGE 1:** fever, headache, light sensitivity. **STAGE 2:** (3-4 days) high fever, rash. NOTE: fatalities have been reported.	• ***antibiotics*** (doxycycline)
Tick Paralysis	Leg weakness, progressing to paralysis as long as tick is still attached. Respiratory arrest can occur. Deaths have been reported.	• removal of tick

TICK DISEASE PREVENTION & TICK REMOVAL TECHNIQUE:

• Wear light-colored, long sleeves/pants that are taped and tucked. Check entire body post-outing.
• Unattached ticks on skin can be removed by using the sticky back of duct tape. Attached ticks should be pulled off gently with tweezers and the area then cleansed.
• 0.5% permethrin repellent or DEET® works well (caution with high concentrations of DEET).

NOTES

RESPIRATORY SYSTEM / ASTHMA - 60

ASTHMA

Asthma is a chronic inflammatory disease of the lower airway that presents itself with acute episodes of bronchospasm manifested by respiratory distress, wheezes and persistent cough. Patients who have progressed to severe asthma have a combination of the following: respiratory rate >30 breaths per minute, mental status changes (anxious, fatigued, agitated or combative), or sweats, and are frequently unable to speak in full sentences or lie down.

Mechanism
- Lower airway constriction/swelling

Causes/triggers
- Cold air, environmental irritants (smoke, ozone), exercise, emotional stress, allergens (bee stings, pollens, molds), infection

TREATMENT

- **PROP**

- **If PROP is not working and the patient is not responding to or is unable to use his beta agonist MDI (e.g. albuterol metered dose inhaler), start supplemental oxygen (if possible)**

-**Consider IM injection of epinephrine MDI* 1/1000.**
 (The dose is 0.01 ml/kg body weight to a maximum of 0.3 ml-(suitable for a person over 60 lbs). May be repeated up to two times within 30 minutes if not responding or worsening)
-**Oral or injectable corticosteroids***
 (e.g., prednisone 1mg/kg up to 60mg; dexamthethasone used for HACE may also be used)
-**Once the patient improves, encourage use of MDI**
-**Evacuate**

 * These are prescription drugs and should only be administered by a properly trained and authorized provider.

ASTHMA ASSESSMENT

		MILD	MODERATE	SEVERE
SIGNS	Pulse	<100bpm	100-120bpm	>120bpm
	Wheeze	moderate; often only at end-expiratory	loud; throughout exhalation	inhale/exhale; lung sounds may be diminished
	Use of accessory muscles	usually not	commonly	usually paradoxical chest/abdomen movement
	Resp. rate	increased	increased	often greater than 30 bpm
SYMPTOMS	Mental status	may be agitated	usually agitated	agitated, drowsy or confused
	Talks in...	sentences	phrases	one or two short words
	S.O.B.	• while walking • can lie down	• while talking • prefers to sit	• while at rest • sits upright

ANAPHYLAXIS-62

ANAPHYLAXIS

• Anaphylaxis is a life-threatening allergic reaction that is commonly associated with insect stings, food allergies, and medications.

• Reactions from stings usually occur within a few minutes. Reactions from foods/medicines generally occur within 30 minutes.

• Some patients do not have a prior allergic history. Some who do will not have a subsequent reaction.

• People who die from anaphylaxis generally die from the respiratory compromise. Airway obstruction and vascular collapse are particulary ominous symptoms.

• Signs and symptoms range from minor to severe.

• Evacuate all patients treated for anaphylaxis. Rebound (biphasic reactions) can occur within 24 hrs. Treat like anaphylaxis.

Causes	Evaluation/S/Sx	Treatment

Ingested or injected antigen
• Bee sting
• Shellfish
• Dairy
• Nuts
• Medicines
• Other
	• Hot, burning skin Sx
	• Hives, red, blotchy skin
	• Respiratory distress
	  (often wheezes)
	• Upper/Lower airway
	  swelling/constriction
	• Anxious, decreasing AVPU
	• Elevated pulse
	• Blood pressure often lowered
		• General respiratory treatment
		• **P** osition of comfort
		  R eassurance
		  O 2 as available
		  P ositive pressure ventilation
		• Epinephrine (SC/IM)*
		  See dosage, pg. 60.
		• Prednisone 60 mg**
		• Oral antihistamines
		  Diphenhydramine 50 mg *
		• Evacuation, consider ALS
		*Adult dosages

 * These are prescription drugs and should only be administered by a properly trained and authorized provider.

CHEST PAIN

Chest pain can often be the result of a serious cardiac event, or it could be from less serious problems such as a broken rib or a respiratory infection. Use of the PAS to determine the cause if possible.

Risk factors that increase the chances of a heart attack include:
Family history, or personal history of heart problems
- increasing age, especially males
- high levels of cholesterol
- high blood pressure
- sedentary lifestyle
- smoking
- diabetes
- obesity

Heart attack signs and symptoms can include:
- chest pain, chest tightness or pressure.
- pain radiating to the jaw and left arm
- weakness, dizziness and lightheadedness
- nausea, vomiting or indigestion, heartburn
- women and men can present different symptoms
- sweating
- shortness of breath

It is difficult in the field to differentiate a simple angina attack from a true heart attack. It is more concerning however if the chest pain:
- occurs during non-stressful events, e.g., sleeping
- is not relieved with rest, or nitroglycerin
- is deemed serious by the patient

Treatment includes:
- arrangements for evacuation and ALS intercept ASAP
- rest, position of comfort
- oxygen
- **nitroglycerine** *(patients with a history of angina will often carry this medication)*
- **aspirin** *(if not allergic)*

As a general rule, these patients should not walk out unless it is absolutely necessary, and their chest pain has resolved.

DIABETES - 64

DIABETES

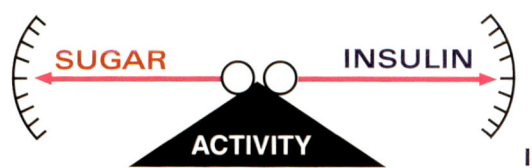

SUGAR:
Primary energy source

INSULIN:
Allows cells to use sugar for energy

Diabetics do not produce enough insulin to balance the sugar/energy needs of their bodies. Some must take insulin (injectable) or oral agents to control their diabetes, others control with diet. The wilderness environment can pose additional challenges to the diabetic's ability to balance activity and insulin vs. sugar levels.

Tips to help diabetics in the wilderness include:

• Diabetics should monitor blood sugar frequently when in the wilderness. Someone else in the party should also know how to operate their glucose tester. Keep accurate records of blood sugar levels. Check blood sugar before peak effects of medication (regular insulin peaks at 4 hrs, intermediate at 8 hrs, oral agents depend on the medication).
• Meals should be planned with as much routine as possible.
• Have food and water available and encourage frequent munching.
• Have a backup source of insulin and perhaps injectable glucagon available. Glucagon is an injectable emergency medicine used to stimulate the release of glucose in a hypoglycemic patient. The diabetic should be able to teach you when and how to do this if needed.
• Diabetics are more prone to hypothermia, frostbite and wound infections.
• Short term problems include: hypoglycemia (too low blood sugar) and hyperglycemia (too high blood sugar). Long term problems include heart disease, vision problems, circulatory problems, kidney failure and infections.
• Check feet frequently for blisters or cuts. Aggressive wound management is indicated to avoid infection.
• Illnesses can be much more serious with diabetics. Fever, any infection, significant vomiting, diarrhea and/or decreased ability to maintain food and water intake are indications for evacuation.

DIABETES

	Hypoglycemia	Hyperglycemia
Mechanism	• Caused by an imbalance of supply and demand, such as not eating enough an/or an increase in caloric needs (e.g. exercise, shivering) • Insulin levels are usually OK, but it can occasionally be caused by too much insulin • High risk times are during long hard days, in the middle of the night and times of peak action of the medication.	• Insufficient insulin levels • Too much food intake without burning it off (e.g. stuck in a base camp, waiting out a storm) • Significant dehydration, caused by kidneys attempting to get rid of extra sugar through increasing urine output (urinary frequency, thirst, headache) • Electrolyte imbalances and acidosis • Body resorts to alternative fuel source (fats) and this makes the problem worse
Assessment	• Rapid onset (minutes, hours) • Mental status changes (irritable, confused, sluggish, slurred speech) followed by a decrease in AVPU • Vital signs often show an adrenaline-like response (vital signs elevated, skin cool and moist, anxiety) • Nighttime hypoglycemia may be evidenced by unusual fatigue, morning headache, and nightmares	• Slow onset (days) • Progressive dehydration • Loss of appetite, nausea • Intense thirst • Flushed, dry skin (usually) • Eventual decrease in mental status and AVPU (very serious) • Possible fruity smell on patient's breath
Treatment	• If patient is unconscious, rub sugar (honey works well) under the tongue and around gums • Oral sugar, ALS, IV Dextrose 50% (D50) • Following the sugar, encourage intake of complex carbohydrates and hydration • Make attempts to prevent recurrence • No need for evacuation unless problem is recurrent, or patient refuses to modify behavior	• Adequate fluid replacement • If only mildly symptomatic (e.g., urine frequency), the patient may be able to make insulin and dietary adjustment based on blood sugar monitoring. • With other symptoms like nausea and vomiting, evacuate for definitive care • Volume loss and electrolyte imbalances can make corrections in the field difficult and dangerous

DIABETES - 65

COMMON MEDICAL PROBLEMS, ASSESSMENT AND TREATMENT

- This is a brief summary of some problems encountered on an extended outing. One should seek the advice of a physician and read up on specific problems that could be encountered.

- Authorization to dispense prescription medicines may need to be obtained.

- Most, if not all, medical problems can be prevented with proper education, preparation, training and attitude. The following HEALTH acronym may help:

Hygiene - Allow time for this. Latrine facilities (with paper) are very important. Make sure participants are using proper techniques in the kitchen for food and H20 handling.

Eating - Adequate nutrition is essential. A radical change in diet may be unappealing to some participants. Have options. Frequent munching is a good approach.

Attitude - Have an open mind; be flexible and patient. Things don't always work the way they should. Have backup plans. Communication among the group is essential.

Limitations - Know the limits of the group. Excessive fatigue is a major contributing factor to minor and serious problems. Modify the objectives, if need be, according to weather, terrain, etc.

Training and fitness- Get fit before the trip. Overuse syndromes, muscle aches, and injuries are a much greater possibility for the unfit.

Hydration - Use urine output as a guide. Hydration is essential for adequate performance and elimination of waste.

COMMON MEDICAL PROBLEMS

- Emphasis should be on prevention and early intervention. Treatment can be supportive, symptomatic or definitive.(NOTE: Field treatment is definitive in many cases.)
- Medications may mask underlying problems and, if not used properly, can worsen the situation. Seek education. Do not over-medicate.
- Be sure to check for allergies before giving medicines.
- Discontinue any medicine if an adverse reaction occurs or if conditions worsen, plus consider evacuation if no improvement within 12-24 hours.
- No medicines are safe during pregnancy unless a physician has okayed them.
- Do not initiate treatment if you are in doubt about what you are treating. Consult a physician if possible.
- All medicines and dosages are given for adults. Consult a physician for pediatric indications and dosages
- Medications should be given orally, unless otherwise stated.
- Of the medicines listed in this reference, there may be alternatives that a physician could prescribe.
- Make sure the med kit is water-tight, protected from impact and thievery.

Problem	Evaluation/Assessment	Treatment
EARS: *FOREIGN BODIES*	Dirt, insects.	• don't probe or jab • mineral oil may help • for insects, shine light into ear to coax them out
EXTERNAL OTITIS *(Swimmer's Ear)*	• ear pain, tenderness of the outer ear • red, swollen canal	• irrigate with Swimmer's Ear® or a dilute acetic acid/ alcohol solution • Antibiotic ear drops (pg. 88)

COMMON MEDICAL PROBLEMS-67

COMMON MEDICAL PROBLEMS-68

Problem	Evaluation/Assessment	Treatment
EARS(cont'd) *OTITIS MEDIA* (middle ear infection)	• significant earache • fever, possible balance problems • most of these are viral and will clear up on their own	• pain medication • start antibiotics with fever, worsening pain or cold symptoms; also if a hx of recurrent infections
EYES: *FOREIGN BODIES*	• pt. usually feels something in his/her eye • irritation, redness, tearing is common • examine corners of eye and under lids	• dab object off the eye with moist gauze • gently irrigate with clean H₂O
CORNEAL ABRASION (scratch to eye)	• similar s/sx as for foreign bodies • persistent irritation and pain	• ophthalmic antibiotics(see pg. 75) • remove foreign body if present • patch eye for 24 hours, if more comfortable
CONJUNCTIVITIS (pinkeye)	• infection to eye; pus drainage, "glued" shut, redness, itching, photosensitive	• antibiotic ointment • do not patch eye(s)
IMPALED OBJECT	• Assess for other injuries. • Determine object depth, angle.	• stabilize object, if possible • patch both eyes
SOLAR KERATITIS (snow blindness)	• delayed onset of severe eye pain • light sensitivity, tearing	• ophthalmic ointment(see pg. 75) • patch eye(s) • pain medications
NOSE: *NOSEBLEEDS*	• causes include trauma, irritation, dry air, hypertension • may be minimal or severe	• sit patient upright • blow out clots • pinch nostrils x 15 min.
IRRITATION (raw nose)	• usually caused by dry air, runny nose • raw inflammation inside nose	• Vaseline® (or similar ointment) inside nose to keep moist

COMMON MEDICAL PROBLEMS

Problem	Evaluation/Assessment	Treatment
TEETH: *TOOTHACHE*	• evaluate dental hygiene, status, history • check for cavities, abscess, trauma	• anesthetic gel (see pg. 74) • oral analgesics (pg. 73) • oil of clove, Orabase®, Numzit® • antibiotics if infected
LOST FILLING OR CHIPPED TOOTH	Assess for other injuries.	• rinse with clean water • Cavit® or Orabase® w/ benzocaine
TOOTH KNOCKED OUT	Find it, clean it, and if intact	• cover with dental wax Replace tooth in socket, • evacuate
DENTAL ABSCESS	Swelling, pain, fever.	• warm compresses, evacuate • pain meds, antibiotics (pg. 75)
RESPIRATORY PROBLEMS: *SORE THROAT*	• Throat feels raw, hard to swallow. • Possible infection showing red or white blotches in back of mouth. • fever, swollen glands, pus drainage	• pain meds, fever reduction • gargle with warm saltwater • lozenges (Cepacol®) • if infection, antibiotics
UPPER RESPIRATORY INFECTION:(URI) Cold, flu	• Viral infection with congestion, runny nose, body aches, possible low-grade fever, sore throat.	• rest • maintain hydration, clear fluids • pain meds, decongestants
LOWER RESPIRATORY INFECTION: - bronchitis - pneumonia	• Chest cold, weakness, fever, chills, productive cough, coughing colors, wheezing • Pleuritic chest pain.	• rest, fluids • pain/fever meds • expectorant (loosens chest fluids) • oral antibiotics
DRY COUGH	• Dry, non-productive, hacking cough causes: altitude, dry air, irritants	• throat lozenges • cough suppressants (at night)

Problem	Evaluation/Assessment	Treatment
RESPIRATORY (cont'd)		
ASTHMA	• Pt. often has history of asthma and can identify cause and give self-treatment. • Pt. is often anxious with elevated vital signs. • If asthma progresses - ↓ AVPU, cyanosis, severe respiratory distress.	• remove cause of asthma if possible • position of comfort, reassurance • O2, PPV if needed/available (ALS) • inhaler - 2 puffs albuterol • epinephrine if severe - .5 mg SC
GASTROINTESTINAL PROBLEMS:		
ABDOMINAL PAIN	Abdominal pain can be difficult to assess in any context. General guidelines for assessment include minor vs. serious; field fix vs. evacuate; casual evac. vs. ALS intercept. Use the **ABDOMINAL** acronym: ***A****SSOCIATED S/SX* - Nausea/vomiting, fever, weakness, headache. ***B****LOOD* - In stool/vomit: how much? when? red or tarry black? ***D****ESCRIPTION* - Sharp vs dull; comes in waves vs. constant; localized vs. general; does it radiate? Is it worsening? ***O****NSET* - When did it start? Slow onset, or sudden? What makes it better or worse? ***M****ENSTRUAL HX* - Cycle normal, missed period, cramps, pregnancy? ***I****NSPECTION/PALPATION* - Look at abdomen; palpate for tenderness 4 quadrants ***N****UTRITION/HYDRATION* - Have they been eating/drinking; peeing + pooping? ***A****USCULTATION* -Active, hyperactive or quiet bowel sounds? ***L****OSING VOLUME?* - Vomiting, diarrhea - How much? Volume status.	• Treat the underlying problem if possible and, if dehydrated, give oral or IV fluids • Consider evacuation with any of the RED FLAGS: - fever, especially if high - dehydrated, volume shock - persistent vomiting >24 hr. - diarrhea >24 hr. - blood in vomit/stool (other than a small amount i.e., hemorrhoid - persistent pain, tenderness (again, no more than 24 hr) - abdominal trauma - pregnancy (even remotely possible - altered mental status • Specific treatments to follow.

COMMON MEDICAL PROBLEMS-70

GASTROINTESTINAL PROBLEMS (cont'd):

Problem	Evaluation/Assessment	Treatment
NAUSEA/VOMITING	• Cause may be benign (anxiety) or may be caused by motion sickness, food poisoning, G.I. infections, flu, and more. • Most n/v is self-limited & will resolve within 24 hours. • A limited bout of vomiting is not dangerous; symptomatic relief is appropriate, observe for any red flags	• If pt. is dehydrated, give sips of water & electrolytes; use urine output as a guide. IV volume may be appropriate. • Motion/sea sickness: stop cause if possible. -Antihistamines (diphenhydramine) 25-50mg every 4-6 hours -Phenergan 25mg every 4-6 hours -Pepto-Bismol®
ACID STOMACH, HEARTBURN, ULCER; INDIGESTION	• Epigastric pain may be relieved by eating. • Use pt. hx to evaluate severity.	• Antacids: Mylanta®, Rolaids® • Anti-ulcer meds; famotidine (Pepcid®)20mg daily, or omeprazole (Prilosec®)20mg daily
DIARRHEA (loose, watery stool) **PREVENTION:** -cook food completely -purify all water -peel own fruits/vegetables -bottled or purified H20 - avoid milk	• Most diarrhea is self-limited & will resolve within 24 hours. • Use ABDOMINAL assessment & red flags to guide evacuation decision. • Volume depletion is the major concern. • Use PAS, exam, vitals, Hx to identify cause. • Giardia (Giardia Lamblia) has a 7-14 day incubation period. Presentation includes abdominal cramps, diarrhea, bloating	• maintain hydration: clear fluids (electrolyte/glucose solution~<5%) • Soothing Agents-PeptoBismol®2 tabs every hour, not to exceed 20 per day • Anti-motility meds (loperamide) Imodium® 4 mg loading then 2 mg every 4 hours, not to exceed 16mg/day • Antibiotics for travelers diarrhea or any G.I. infection • Giardia - (metronidazole) Flagyl® 250mg every 8 hrs for 7-10 days

COMMON MEDICAL PROBLEMS-71

Problem	Evaluation/Assessment	Treatment
GASTROINTESTINAL (cont'd):		
CONSTIPATION *provide opportunity to use latrine*	• Cramping, unable/unwilling to move bowels; hard, dry stool. • Causes include lack of exercise, lack of opportunity to defecate, dehydration	• hydration • laxative: Milk of Magnesia® 1-2 tbsps • caffeine sometimes works • local lubricant; glycerin suppositories • stool softener; Colace 50-100mg
HEMORRHOIDS	• Inflammation, itching, redness to anus. • Pain while defecating. • Possible small amount of blood in stool.	• soothing cream; Anusol® • hydrocortisone cream • Tucks® pads
GENITOURINARY PROBLEMS:		

URINARY TRACT INFECTIONS
(infection of bladder)
 	
PREVENTION:
• *hydration*
• *toilet paper*
• *opportunity:*
  - to urinate
  - for hygiene
	• UTIs occur mostly in women (short urethra)
	• Contributing factors: dehydration, lack of opportunity for personal hygiene, no toilet paper, history of prior problems.
	• S/Sx - painful, burning urination, frequent urge to urinate; often dark colored, blood-tinged urine.
	• **Red Flags** include: back pain/tenderness, high fever, chills. This indicates kidney infection.
		• aggressively maintain hydration
		• cranberry juice (does help for UTI prevention)
		• antibiotics (see pg.75)
		• antibiotic Tx, consider evac consider ALS; push H20

KIDNEY STONES	• Sudden onset of severe, cramping pain radiating from flank to genitals. • nausea, sweating	• strong pain medicine (pg. 73) • push fluids • wait for stone to pass • consider evacuation

Problem	Evaluation/Assessment	Treatment
GENITOURINARY (cont'd):		
VAGINITIS	• Vaginal itching, burning, discharge. Causes include persistent wet/unclean environments, irritation, prior Hx	• anti-fungal cream/suppositories; fluconazole (150mg)(Diflucan®) j PI 0.25% for vaginal douche; terconazole (Terazol®), clotrimazole • cool, dry, clean environment
PAIN	• Pain is a normal response to a problem. Not all pain is bad. • Pain medicines should not be given to anyone who is neurologically impaired. • Use the least potent medicine to do the job, but use enough to relieve the pain. • Be sure to check for allergies.	**THE FOLLOWING MEDICINES AND DOSAGES ARE LISTED FOR ADULTS. CONSULT A PHYSICIAN FOR PEDIATRIC INDICATIONS AND DOSAGES** • **ASPIRIN:** good pain relief, fever reducer, anti-inflammatory (650mg every 4-6 hours). • **ACETAMINOPHEN:** good pain relief, fever reducer, good for people who are sensitive to aspirin (650 mg every 4-6 hours). • **IBUPROFEN OR OTHER NSAIDs:** excellent pain relief, fever reducer, anti-inflammatory (400-600 mg every 4-6 hours, not to exceed 2400mg/24hours). • **HYDROCODONE (RX);** for significant pain, cough suppressant (5 mg 1-2 every 4-6 hours - sold in combination with either acetaminophen (Lortab®) or ibuprofen)

COMMON MEDICAL PROBLEMS-73

SKIN + SOFT TISSUE:

Problem	Evaluation/Assessment	Treatment
ITCHING:	Bug bites, rash, heat, irritants.	• hydrocortisone cream 1/2-1% • Diphenhydramine (Benadryl®) 25-50 mg every 4-6 hours • Hydroxyzine hydrochloride (Atarax®) 25-50mg every 8 hours
	Jock itch, athletes foot (itching, peeling of skin, burning).	• clean, dry, well-ventilated, if possible • anti-fungal cream/powder (Tinactin® or Lotromin®) • povidone Iodine (Betadine®)
ALLERGIC REACTIONS: **PREVENTION:** long clothing l-topical barriers (Ivy Shield®, Stokoguard®) -post exposure washes; Technu®, Oak-N-Ivy Cleanser®	• Poison ivy • Sumac • Poison oak • red, itchy, blistered skin	• drying agents (Prax®, Calamine®, Sarna®) • Topical steroids; (hydrocortisone cream 1/2 - 1%) • oral steroids if severe; Prednisone Rx 60 mg/day for 7-10 days • anti-itch meds; Diphenhydramine Benadryl® (25-50 mg every 4-6 hours)
SKIN INFECTIONS:	• **LOCAL** - red, swollen, tender pus • **SYSTEMATIC** - pain, red streak, fever, enlarged lymp nodes, increased pain, blistering, looks sick	• **LOCAL** - rest, elevatem warm water soaks, encourage pus to drain • **SYSTEMATIC** - above plus antibiotics; consider evacuation, may need surgical drainage

ANTISEPTIC SOLUTIONS FOR THE SKIN:
- **Povidone Iodine (Betadine®)** 10% for topical use; dilute to 1% for wound cleaning.
- **ANESTHETIC GEL** *(available in 5 ml tube)*:
- **Lidocaine 2%** - numbs the area so that proper cleaning and debridement can occur. Leave on 5-10 minutes prior to cleaning. Do not use on > 5% Total Body Surface Area (TBSA). Do not repeat use.

Antibiotic	Dose	Uses/Indications	Precautions
CEPHALEXIN (Keflex®)	250 mg every 6 hours for 7-10/Days	• skin & wound infections • upper & lower respiratory infections • urinary tract infections • ear infections	• Do not use if pt. has a Hx of severe penicillin(PCN) reactions; use levofloxacin instead.
AMOXICILLIN/ CLAVULANIC ACID (Augmentin®)	875 mg twice/day	• skin & wound infections, upper & lower respiratory infections, ear infections, tooth abscesses, mammalian bite	• can cause significant diarrhea • do not use if penicillin allergic
LEVOFLOXACIN (Levoquin®)	250-500 mg once/day	• UTI (7-10 days) • skin infections (5-20 days) • G.I. infections, traveler's diarrhea (3-5 days) • use TMP/SMX® (see below) as a substitute	• dizziness, GI, insomnia stop if tendon pain develops
TRIMETHOPRIM SULFA-METHOXAZOLE (TMP/SMX D. S.®, Bactrim®,Septra®)	1 tab every 12 hours	• G.I. infections (3-5 D) • UTI (7-10 D) • ear infections	• Do not use if allergic to sulfa drugs
CORTISPORIN otic drops	2-3 drops in ear 4 times/day for 7 days	• external ear infections	• Keep ear dry if possible
ERYTHROMYCIN ointment	Apply to inner surface of lid.	• eye infection (conjunctivitis).. • solar keratitis (snow blindness)............... • corneal abrasion............	• Do not patch eye(s) • Do patch eye(s) • Do patch eye(s)

COMMON MEDICAL PROBLEMS-75

COMMON MEDICAL PROBLEMS - 76

WATER DISINFECTION

BOILING:

Contrary to popular belief, bringing water to a boil at any elevation will kill all pathogens that could cause illness*. Boiling does not remove chemicals, however.

*Wilderness Medical Society position papers

FILTERS:

Most filters do remove protozoans, cysts, bacteria and parasitic eggs. They do not remove viruses, as a rule. Iodine resin filters do kill viruses. Check the manufacturers instructions and guidelines

CHEMICAL DISINFECTANTS:

Iodine and chlorine. These techniques approach 100% removal of all living organisms. Contact time must be lengthened when using in cold water and the dose must be increased in cloudy, dirty water. Most authorities prefer iodine over chlorine. Halogen does not remove/kill cryptosporidium. Do not flavor treated water until contact time has elapsed.

AMOUNT NEEDED IN 1 QT. TO YIELD:			
	4 PPM	**8 PPM**	NOTE:
Iodine tablets	1/2 tab	1 tab	• Pre-filter water before treatment.
2 % Iodine Tincture	5 drops	10 drops	• Flavor water only after treat-
10% P.I. solution	8 drops	16 drops	ment time is complete.
Iodine crystals	13 ml	26 ml	• 1 drop = 1gtt = .05 ml
Halizone tabs	2 tabs	4 tabs	
Household bleach	2 drops	4 drops	

	WATER TEMP.	**4PPM**	**8PPM**
CONTACT TIME NEEDED FOR			
VARIOUS CONCENTRATIONS	40° F/5° C	180 min	60 min
AND WATER TEMPERATURES	59° F/15° C	60 min	30 min
NEEDED TO KILL ORGANISMS:	86°F/30° C	45 min	15 min

NOTES

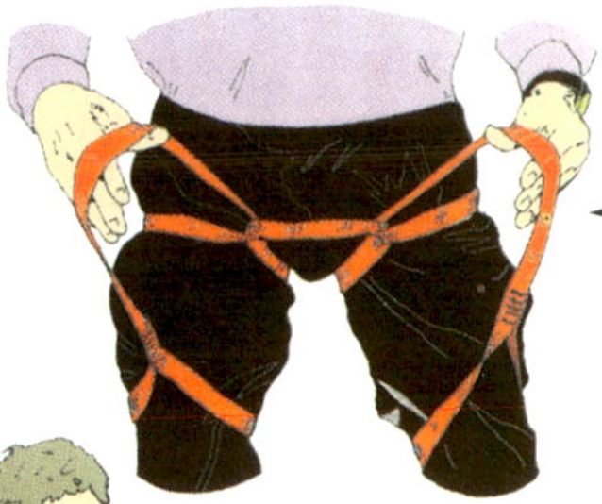

PATIENT CARRIES-78

Place on patient

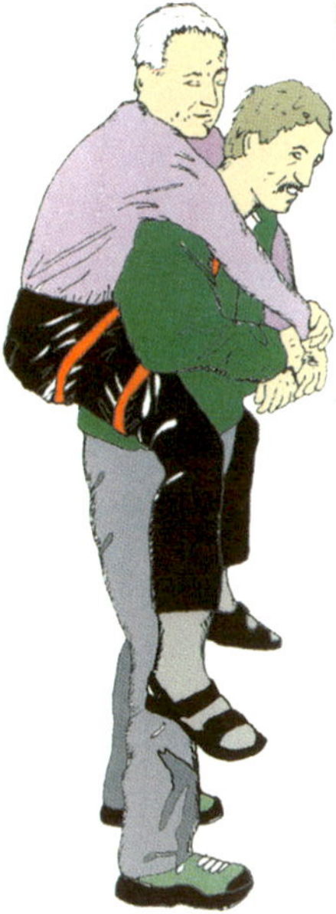

Wear patient like a backpack

Piggyback Carry

using elephant ears.
Make a bight with the center of the webbing and put on patient as per #1 and #2 on previous patient carry example. Slip patient's legs through end loops of elephant ears to create shoulder straps. Put patient on your back like a backpack. (Note: to protect yourself from injury, it may be necessary to walk with ski poles or helpers on each side for stability and support.) Be sure to pad under shoulder straps.

- Some victims can be safely carried out of the wilderness in an upright position. Obviously the weight of the victim is a consideration as well as the strength of the rescuers.
- A 20' length of webbing works well.
- Rescuers should pad shoulders (underneath webbing) for comfort.

PATIENT CARRIES-79

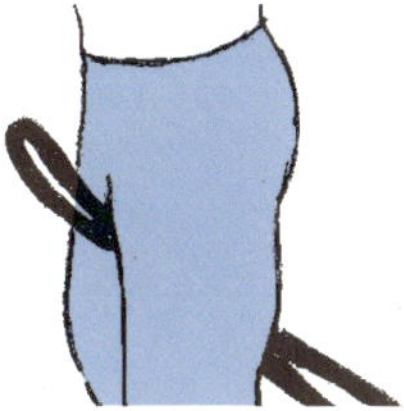

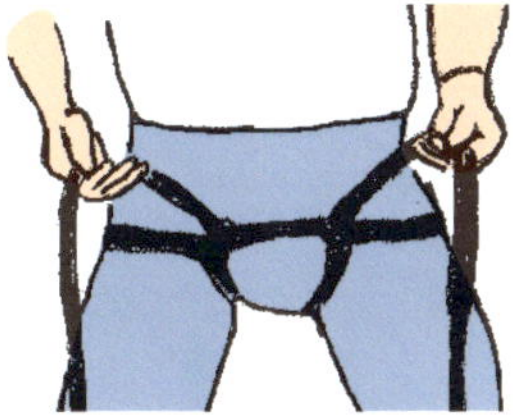

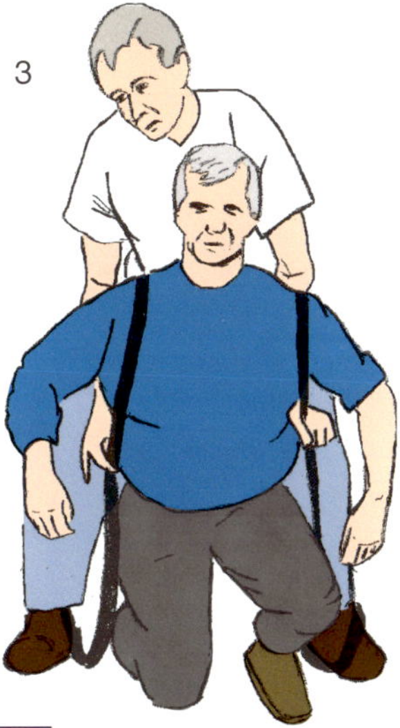

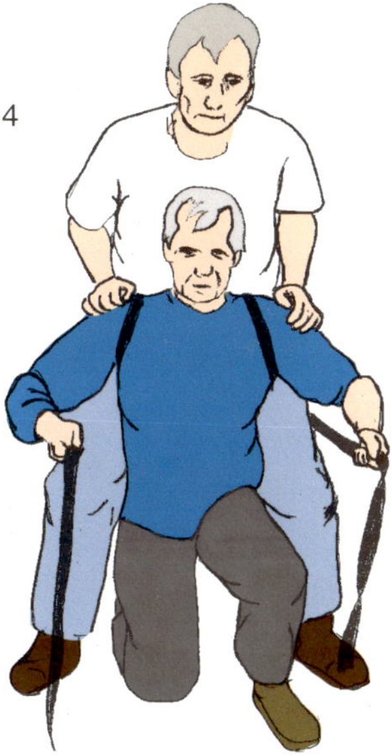

PATIENT CARRIES-80

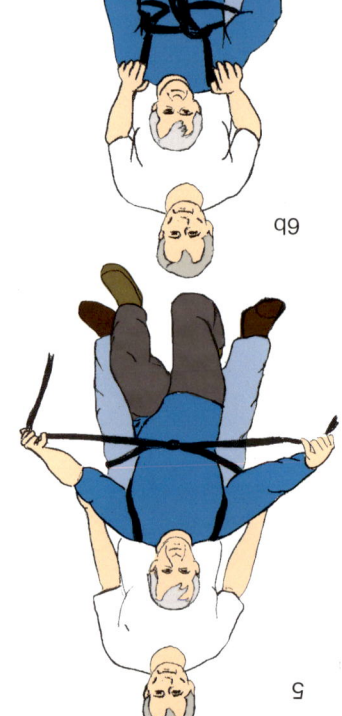

5

6a

6b

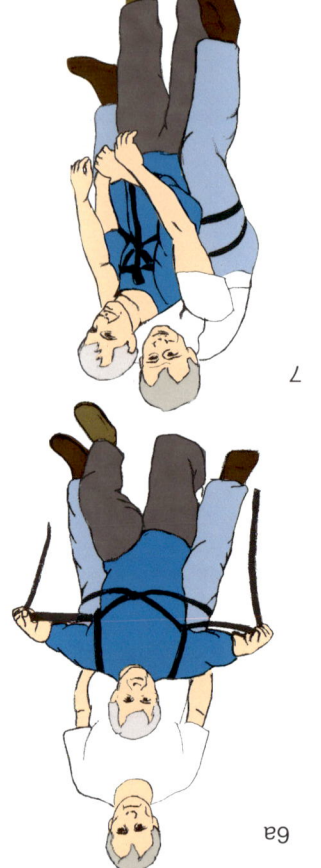

7

SPINE INJURY MANAGEMENT

The spine injured patient should be log-rolled or lifted onto the device. They should be insulated, relatively comfortable and should not shift side to side or end to end.

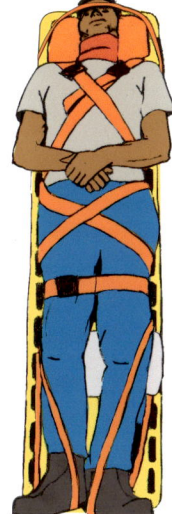

soft head pads

"x" across the torso works well, should anchor shoulders

pads under knees

foot stirrups prevent pt. from sliding down

CERVICAL COLLAR OPTIONS
A: Manufactured

1. Philly Collar®
2. Stiff Neck®
3. 4-Way Quick Collar®

B: Improvised

1. SAM Splint®
2. Ensolite pad(s)
3. Blanket roll

"Tootsie Rolls" may be needed on side of patient to be sure they are **FLUSH** with the sides.

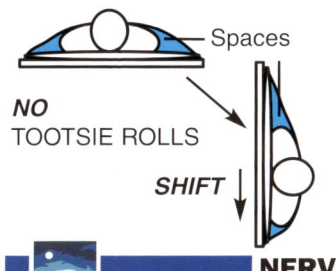

NO TOOTSIE ROLLS
SHIFT

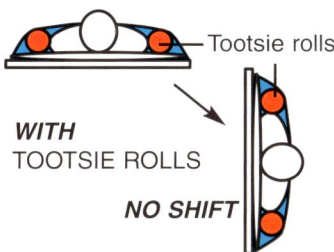

WITH TOOTSIE ROLLS
NO SHIFT

NERVOUS/SPINE INJURY MGMT-81

NERVOUS/SPINE IMMOBILIZATION - 82

Spinal Immobilization - "D ring" strap method

Strap One - Start high on chest, thread through backboard behind armpit. Wrap over shoulder and down across chest.

Strap One - should extend down to PELVIC WINGS. Thread through backboard and bring directly across pelvis. Thread and bring diagonally to opposite shoulder. Then go under the arm and thread the buckle on the chest.

Strap Two - should extend in "box X" pattern from lower pelvis to mid lower leg, with the center of the "X" over the knees.

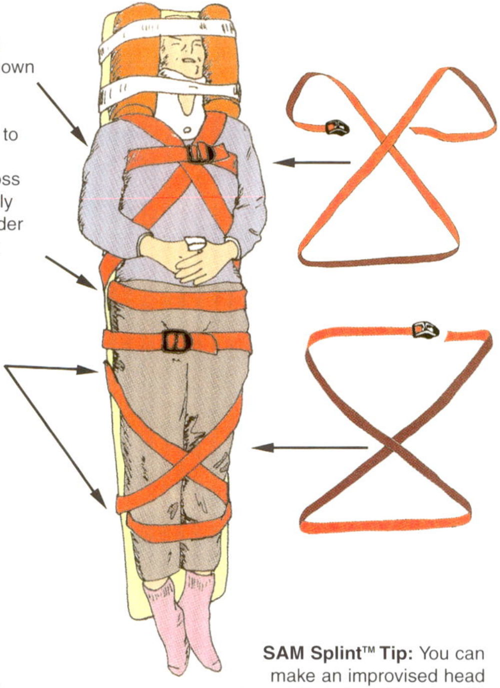

SAM Splint™ Tip: You can make an improvised head immobilizer by folding a SAM Splint™ in thirds, bending and taping

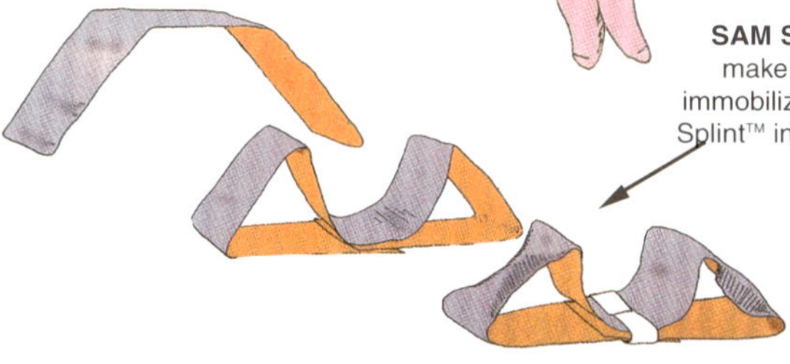

Training and practice are essential.

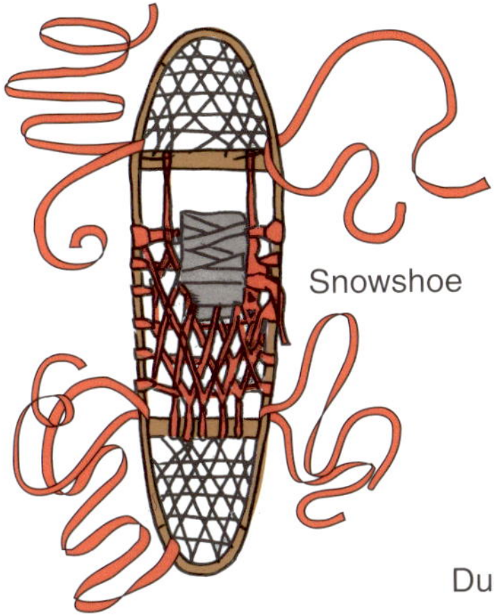

Snowshoe

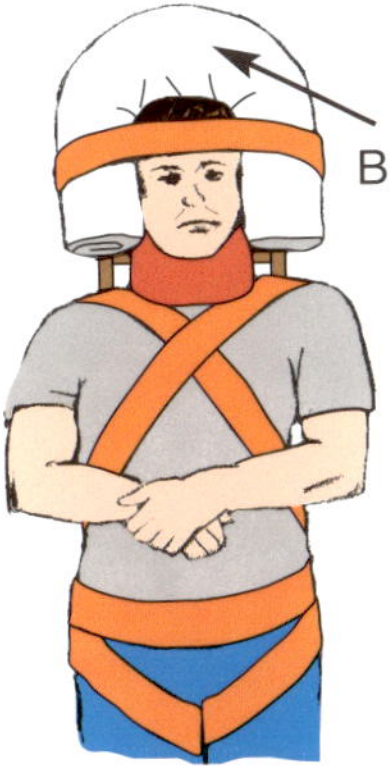

Blanket roll

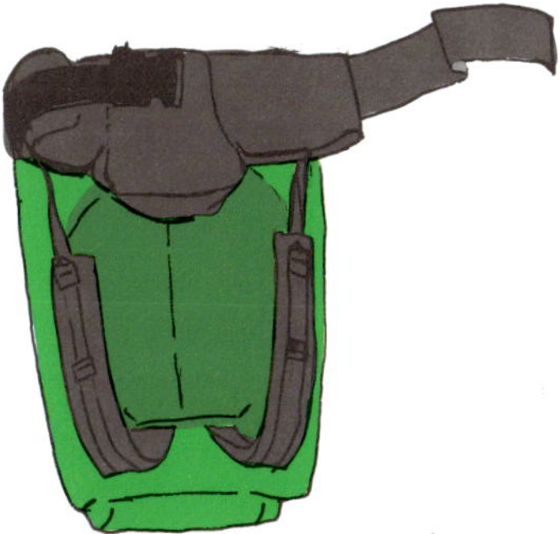

Duct tape

≈ 2.5'

≈ 1.5'

Upside down back-pack

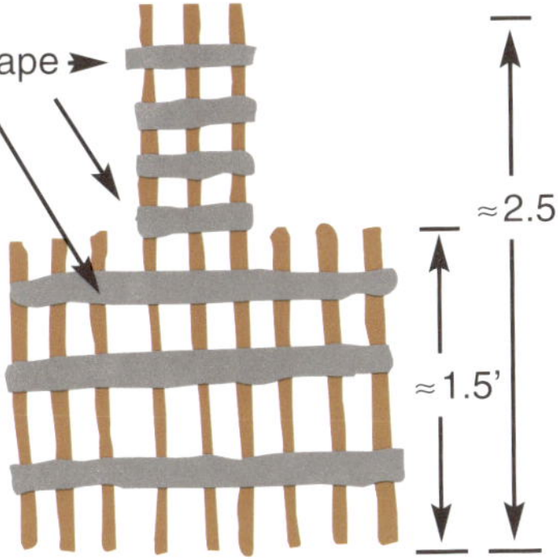

Sticks, tent poles, aluminum stays: tied or taped

IMPROVISED EXTRICATION DEVICES - Vest type
NOTE: These could be used in conjunction with an improvised litter to carry out the spine injured patient.

   **IMPROV. SPINE IMMOBILIZATION-83**

IMPROVISED LITTERS/STRETCHERS-84

Basic stick & rope stretcher (Figs. 1,2)

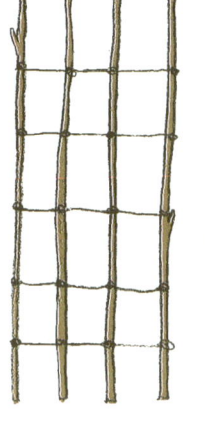

Fig. 1
Rope could be
knotted using
clove hitches.
(Should be
roughly 4' x 6'.)

Fig. 2
Sticks should be
on top of ropes

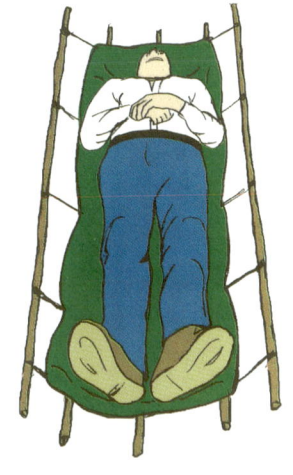

Rigid pole
litter
(Figs. 3,4)

A mattress can be made by stuffing leaves, pine boughs,
or the like into a sleeping bag or tarp.

Paddle and life jacket stretcher: jacket sleeves, etc.

Frame pack stretcher: 3-4 packs needed, connect with hose clamps or lashing string

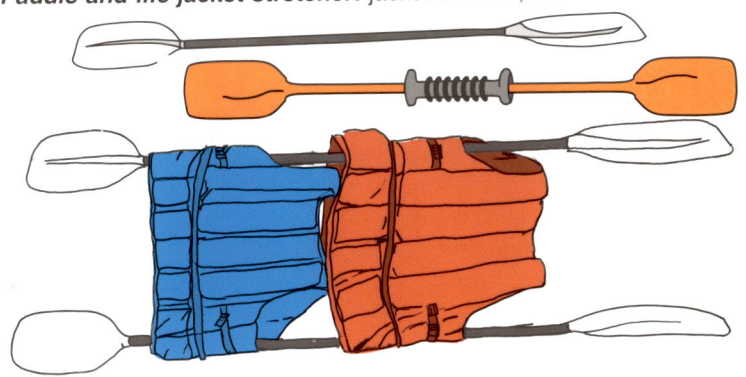

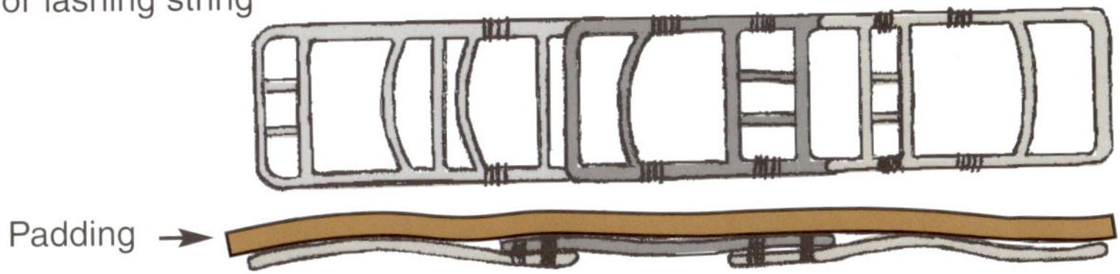

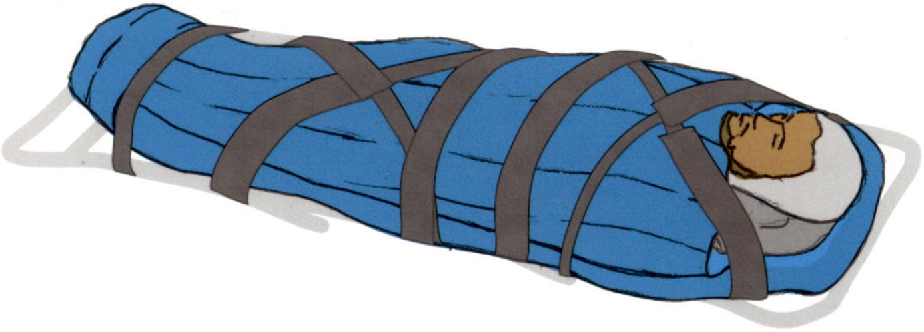

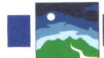

IMPROVISED LITTERS/STRETCHERS-85

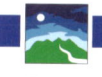 **IMPROVISED LITTERS/STRETCHERS-86**

DELUXE DAISY CHAIN - STICK FRAME LITTER

Materials needed:
- rope; at least 50 feet
- tarp, tent fly
- stick & rope frame (see pg. 29)
- sleeping bags, ensolite pads

STEP 1

Lay out the daisy chain.
6-7' long, arms width, about 15 - 20 "loops"

STEP 2

Put stick & rope frame on daisy chain
Lay padding on the frame and package the patient.
NOTE: An improvised extrication device can be incorporated into this system. (see pg. 83)

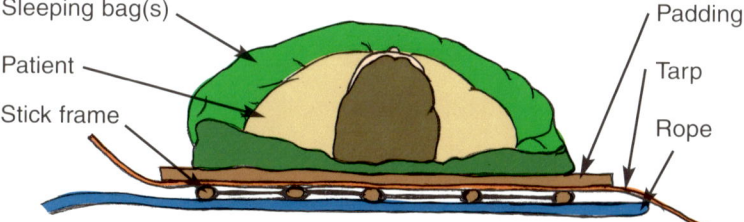

Sleeping bag(s)

Patient

Stick frame

Padding

Tarp

Rope

STEP 3

Tie a loop knot in the end of the rope (i.e. figure 8 on a bite)

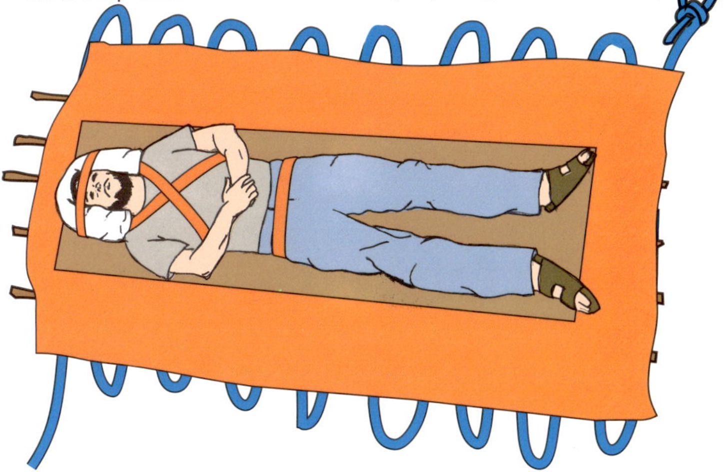

STEP 4

Wrap the patient, cinch and loop the rope up the patient toward the head, then tie off the rope.

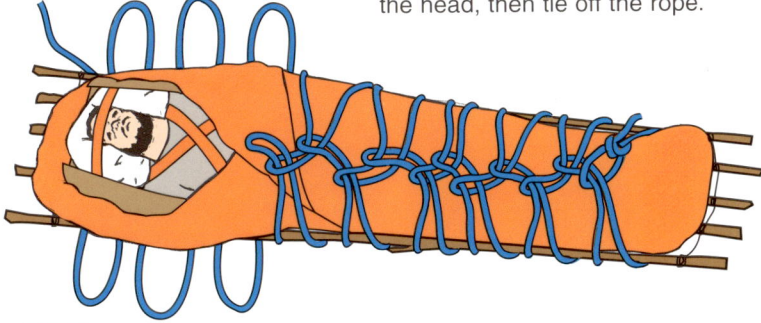

 IMPROVISED LITTERS/STRETCHERS-87

IMPROVISED LITTERS/STRETCHERS-88

SIMPLE TARP STRETCHER

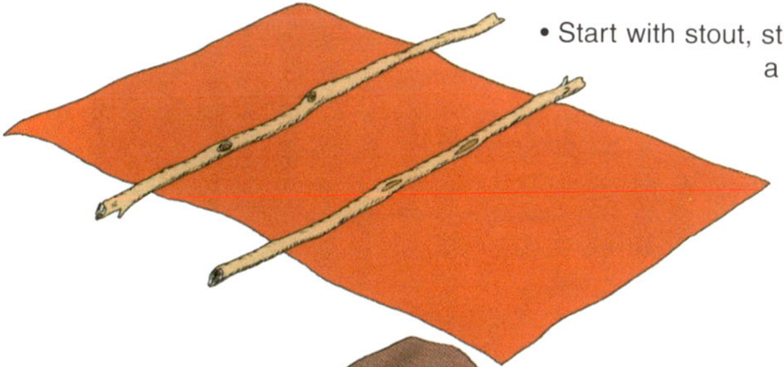

• Start with stout, sturdy poles and a blanket or tarp

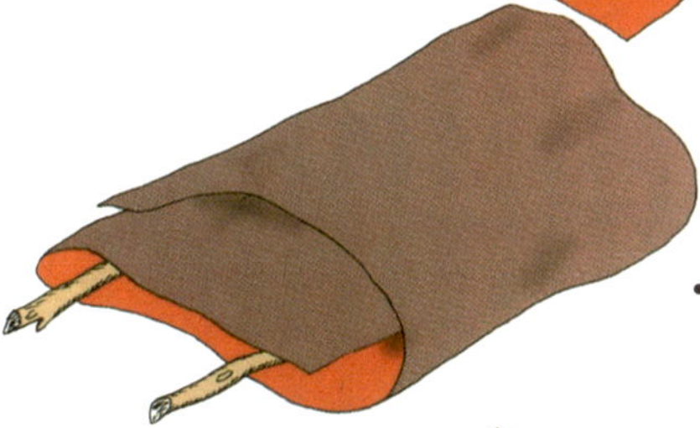

• Fold the blanket/tarp into thirds, making sure that each side extends over the edge of the poles

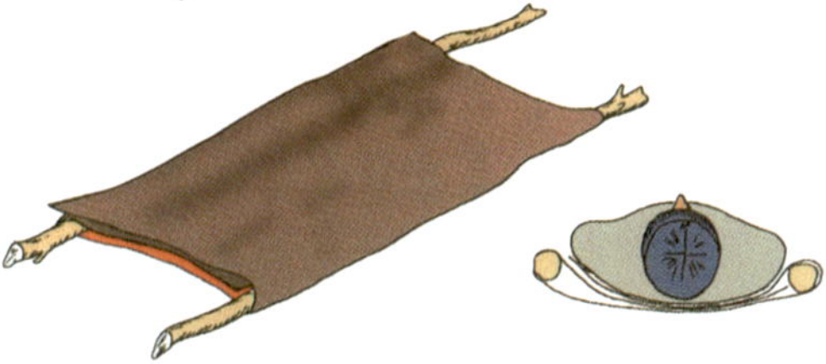

• The weight of the patient's body will pin the blanket/tarp in place

MEDICAL/RESCUE KIT

This is a partial list only, and should be expanded, contracted or modified to meet the many variables expected.

EMERGENCY KIT

PERSONAL PROTECTION
- gloves, mask, eye protection
- pocket mask, one way valve

ASSESSMENT TOOLS
- scissors
- stethoscope
- thermometer (hi/low)
- headlamp
- SOAP forms

OTHER
- heat/cold packs
- ALS supplies as needed/authorized
- blanket pins
- Sawyer Extractor®

EMERGENCY MEDS:
- epinephrine (anaphylaxis)
- altitude meds
- respiratory/cardiac meds
- pain, wound care

TRAUMA CARE
- dressings(sm, med, lg)
- roller gauze
- cravats
- Sam splint(s)®
- oral, nasal airways
- 60 cc syringe (suction/irrigation)

ROUTINE KIT

MEDS
- pain
- respiratory/circulatory
- GI/GU
- HEENT
- skin/wounds
- antibiotics

SUPPLIES
- bandaids
- gloves
- tape, scissors
- sm dressings
- blanket pins
- steri strips
- Spenco® adhesive knit
- Spenco® second skin
- needles/tweezers
- povidone iodine
- Burn Gel®

PERSONAL CARE KIT

Carried by each individual for minor problems, personal needs and preventative measures.

- pain meds
- foot care
- personal meds
- blister care
- toilet paper
- teeth care
- throat lozenges
- lip protection
- eye protection
- sunscreen
- insect repellent
- water disinfectant supplies

MEDICAL/RESCUE KITS-89

SIGNALING/SURVIVAL/RESCUE KIT-90

SIGNALING /SURVIVAL /RESCUE KIT:

- strobe light
- tarp/bivy sack
- flagging tape
- candles, lighter(s)
- duct tape
- whistle
- smoke flares
- water purification tablets
- chemical heat packs
- emergency food (MRE)

- signal mirror
- Cyalume® light sticks
- folding saw
- radio in chest harness, batteries
- meteor flares
- parachute cord, rope
- map/compass
- headlamp(s)
- waterproof paper/pens

OTHER ITEMS TO CONSIDER FOR A "24 HR" PACK

- sturdy backpack (internal frame)
- ensolite pad or Thermarest®
- lightweight sleeping bag
- bivy sack or tarp
- medical / rescue kit
- appropriate clothes/layers:
  - synthetic or wool underwear
  - insulating layers (pile)
  - wind, water proof shells
  - neck, head, eye protection
  - gloves, mitts
  - boots, gators, socks
  - clean change of clothes
    for post-rescue

- food, water
- stove, pot, fuel
- altimeter / barometer
- Leatherman-type tool

- specialized equipment:
  - flight suit, ear protection
  - helmet, head lamp
  - PFD, throw ropes
  - harness
  - technical gear:
    - water
    - cave
    - high angle
  - GPS, cellular phone

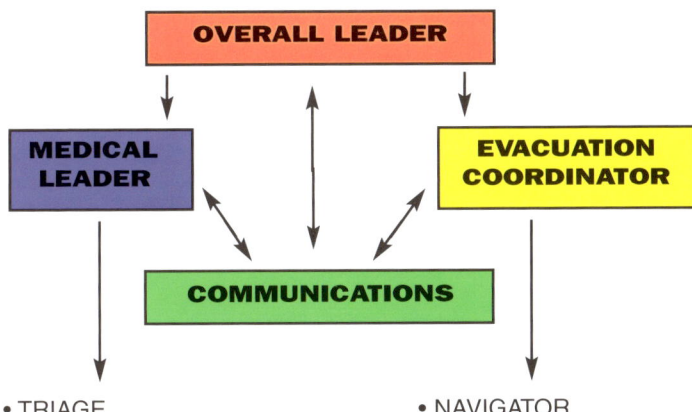

SIGNALING/SURVIVAL/RESCUE KIT-92

HELICOPTER RESCUE AND SAFETY:

- Helicopter rescue can be a great asset, but it is also risky and expensive.
- Consider ground crew training and pre-set protocols within med-evac services.

Helicopter rescue is generally considered when:

1. The victim's chances of recovery are better with air evacuation.
2. A ground evacuation would be unduly long, arduous or dangerous.
3. The number of ground crew is limited.
4. The pilot, crew and helicopter are within their limitations and protocols.

Most pilots will not fly under these conditions:

1. Winds are over 70 km/hr (40 mph) or there are severe gusts.
2. Night flights into mountainous areas.
3. Low visibility (fog, smoke).
4. Poor or unknown landing conditions.
5. Slopes of more than 10°.

Important safety rules:

1. Never approach the helicopter until signaled to do so by the pilot or crewmember.
2. Keep in full view of the pilot and crew.
3. Stay clear of landing zone (LZ) and clear away debris prior to helicopter arrival.
4. Communicate by radio to give pilot local conditions.
5. Stay clear of tail rotor. NOTE: Some helicopters load from the rear. Follow instructions from the crew.

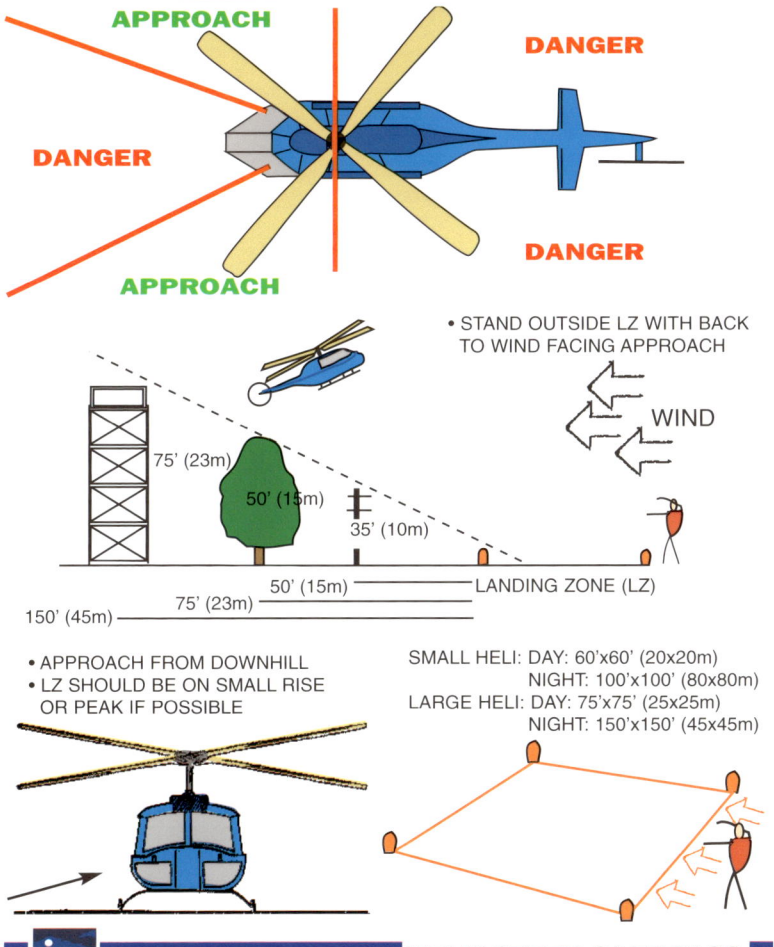

MCI/TRIAGE -94

MASS CASUALTY INCIDENT / DISASTER

GOALS

Goal of rescuers -
• prevent further harm to life and limb if possible, while still protecting rescuers
• attempt to do the greatest amount of good for the greatest number of people
• categorize patients by treatment priority (use triage color system below)

MODIFIED PAS FOR MASS CASUALTY INCIDENT / DISASTER

SCENE SIZEUP
• Same as normal PAS

INITIAL ASSESSMENT
• This is a "quick look, quick fix, move on" approach
(do not spend very much time on any one patient)

  NERVOUS SYSTEM
  • AVPU check - if decreased, patient is PRIORITY RED
  • protect spine as needed, if possible (ask bystanders to help)

  RESPIRATORY
  • Open airway, if necessary
  • Quickly assess ventilations - if too fast or too slow, the patient is PRIORITY RED

  CIRCULATORY
  • Stop severe bleeding (bystanders can help) - if it won't stop, patient is PRIORITY RED
  • DO NOT initiate CPR unless there are plenty of resources to go around (unlikely)

FOCUSED HISTORY AND PHYSICAL EXAM
(usually done in the treatment area)

TRIAGE COLOR / PRIORITY SYSTEM

After the initial assessment is done on a patient, assign a treatment priority to him. Once all are categorized, move them to a safe treatment area in order of severity (RED first, etc.) Wait until they are in a safe treatment area before starting the focused history and physical exam.

RED	• immediate transport, highest priority, first ones out • usually Big 3 problems requiring ALS
YELLOW	• delayed transport, may be serious, but can wait some • these patients may get worse over time, bumping them into RED category
GREEN	• minor conditions that can be treated on scene or can self-transport to the hospital (can also help with patient care)
BLACK	• obviously dead or dying from lethal injuries. As a general rule, CPR should not be initiated on people in this category unless the MOI is lightning.

- **ABC** - Airway, breathing, circulation
- **ABDOMINAL** - pain assessment
- **ALS** - Advanced Life Support
- **AMPLE** - history
- **ASA** - Aspirin
- **ASAP** - as soon as possible
- **ASR** - Acute Stress Reaction
- **AVPU** - consciousness spectrum
- **BID** - twice a day
- **BLS** - Basic Life Support
- **c** - with
- **c/o** - complains of
- **CSM** - Circulation, sensation, motor
- **CVA** - Cerebro-vascular accident
- **D** - day
- **D/C** - discontinue
- **DNR** - do not resuscitate
- **DRT** - dead right there
- **EMS** - Emergency Medical Services
- **FB** - foreign body
- **Fx** - fracture
- **GI** - gastrointestinal
- **GV** - genitourinary
- **gtt** - drops, .05 ml
- **H** - Hour
- **HA** - headache
- **HTN** - hypertension
- **Hx** - history - see **AMPLE**
- **IM** - intramuscular
- **ICP** - intracranial pressure
- **IV** - intraveneous
- **kg** - kilogram
- **LOC** - loss of consciousness
- **MAST** - medical anti-shock trousers
- **Mg** - milligram
- **LAST** - locate, access, stabilize, transport
- **MOI** - mechanism of injury
- **MRE** - meal, ready to eat
- **NTE** - not to exceed
- **N/V** - nausea/vomiting
- **NSAID** - non-steroidal anti-inflammatories
- **O2** - oxygen
- **OTC** - over the counter
- **PAS** - patient assessment system
- **PCN** - penicillin
- **PFA** - pain-free activity
- **PI** - povidone iodine
- **PMH** - past medical history
- **PO** - oral
- **ppm** - parts per million
- **PPV** - positive pressure ventilation
- **PRN** - as needed
- **PROP** - position, reassurance, O2, PPV
- **Q** - every
- **RICE** - rest, ice, compression, elevation
- **ROM** - range of motion
- **Rx** - prescription meds
- **s** - without
- **S/Sx** - signs/symptoms
- **SC** - sub-cutaneous
- **SOB** - short of breath
- **SOAP** - subjective, objective, assessment, plan
- **STOPEATS** - *sugar, T°, O2, pressure, electricity, altitude, toxins, salts*
- **Tbs** - tablespoon
- **TBSA** - total body surface area
- **TID** - three times a day
- **TIP** - traction into position
- **Tx** - treatment
- **URI** - upper respiratory infection
- **UTI** - urinary tract infection
- **VS** - vital signs
- **WBA** - weight bearing ability
- **WNL** - within normal limits
- **WMA** - Wilderness Medical Associates
- *30/30 rule* - proposed as an ideal response to electric storms by the National Lightning Safety Institute

COMMON ABBREV/ACRONYMS-95

INDEX

(*) Indicates additions/changes from present Field Guide version.

A
Abbreviations 95
Acronyms 95
Acute mountain sickness (AMS) .. 54, 55
Airway 4
Allergy 62, 74
Altitude 54, 55
Alveoli 21
Anaphylaxis 62
Angina 63
Ankle
 - evaluation 33
 - treatment 33
Antibiotics 75
*Arterial gas embolus (AGE) .. 51
Arthropods 56
ASR 22
Asthma 21, 60, 61
AVPU 6

B
Bleeding 40
BLS 7-9
Blisters 42
Blood pressure 11, 23
Burns 41
Breathing 5

C
Cardiogenic shock 22
Cervical collar 81, 82
Circulation 5
Circulatory system 22
Chest pain 63
Chest wall trauma 21
*Collateral ligament 31, 32
Concussion 24
Conjunctivitis 68
Corneal abrasion 68

Constipation 72
Conversions 99
CPR
 -summary 10
 -wilderness 9
*Cruciate ligament 31, 32
CSM 25, 26, 29, 30, 38

D
Daisy chain 98
*Decompression sickness (Bends) .. 51
Dental abcess 69
Diabetes 64, 65
Diarrhea 71
Dislocations
 -evaluation 28-30
 -treatment 28-30
Drowning 50

E
Ears 67
*Emergency rolls 7, 8
Evacuation 78-88
Exam 11
Eyes 68

F
Femur fractures 28, 39
Fractures 25-27
Frostbite 47
Focused Hx, Exam 11

G
Gastrointestinal 70-72
Genitourinary 72, 73

H
*HEALTH 66
Heart attack 63

Heart burn ... 71	Mechanism of injury ... 3
Heat related problems ... 48, 49	Medical kit ... 89
Heat exhaustion ... 48, 49	Medications
Heat stroke ... 48, 49	-altitude ... 55
Helicopter rescue ... 93, 94	-antibiotics ... 75
Hemorrhoids ... 73	-antiseptics ... 74
High altitude cerebral edema (HACE) ... 54, 55	-cardiac ... 63
High altitude pulmonary edema (HAPE) ... 54, 55	-pain ... 73
History (Hx) ... 11	Musculoskeletal
Hot spots ... 42	-evaluation ... 25, 26
Hyperthermia ... 48, 49	-treatment ... 25, 27
Hyponatremia ... 49	

N

Nausea/vomiting ... 71
Near drowning ... 50
Nervous system ... 6, 24
Nosebleeds ... 68

Hypothermia
-assessment ... 44
-packaging ... 45, 46

O

Otitis, externea (swimmer's ear) ... 67

I

Impaled objects ... 40
Improvised
-splints ... 27
-stretchers ... 83-88
Initial assessment ... 4-8
Ingested toxins ... 56
Intracranial pressure (ICP) ... 24
Itching ... 74

P

Patient carries ... 78-80
PAS ... 2-12
Personal care kit ... 89
*PROP ... 5, 21, 22, 24, 50, 51, 55
Pulse ... 11

J
K

Kidney stones ... 72
Knee
 -evaluation ... 31, 32

Q
R

Rabies ... 40
*Radio SOAP ... 12
Respiratory
 -infections ... 69
 -summary ... 21
Rescue team ... 91
RICE ... 25
*Rope litter ... 86, 87

L

Lightning ... 52, 53
Litters ... 35-37, 81-88
Lower airway ... 21, 60, 62
Lyme disease ... 58

M

Marine toxins ... 57
Mass casualty incident (MCI) ... 94

S

Safety/scene ... 3
*SAM splint ... 82, 87
SAMPLE history ... 11

INDEX - 97

INDEX - 98

Scorpions 57
*Scuba diving injuries 51
Seizures 24
Shock
   -cardiogenic 22
   -vascular 22
   -volume 22, 23
Signaling/survival 90
Skin 11, 74
Snake bites 56
SOAP notes 12-29
Solar keratitis (snow blindness) 68
Spiders 57
Spine injury
   -assessment 35
   -treatment 81-88
STOPEATS 21, 24

T
Teeth 69
Tetanus 40
Ticks 58
Toothache 69
Toxins 56-58
Traction splints 38, 39

U
Upper airway 21
Urinary tract infection (UTI) 72

V
Vaginitis 73
Vascular shock 22
Vital signs 11
Volume shock 22, 23

W
Water disinfection 76

X
Y
Z